T0350253

User–Centered Software Development for the Blind and Visually Impaired:

Emerging Research and Opportunities

Teresita de Jesús Álvarez Robles
Universidad Veracruzana, Mexico

Francisco Javier Álvarez Rodríguez
Universidad Autónoma de Aguascalientes, Mexico

Edgard Benítez–Guerrero
Universidad Veracruzana, Mexico

A volume in the Advances in
Systems Analysis, Software
Engineering, and High Performance
Computing (ASASEHPC) Book Series

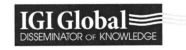

Published in the United States of America by
    IGI Global
    Engineering Science Reference (an imprint of IGI Global)
    701 E. Chocolate Avenue
    Hershey PA, USA 17033
    Tel: 717-533-8845
    Fax: 717-533-8661
    E-mail: cust@igi-global.com
    Web site: http://www.igi-global.com

Library of Congress Cataloging-in-Publication Data

Names: Alvarez Robles, Teresita de Jesus, 1988- editor. | Alvarez
  Rodriguez, Francisco Javier, editor. | Benitez-Guerrero, Edgard, 1972-
  editor.
Title: User-centered software development for the blind and visually impaired
  : emerging research and opportunities / Teresita de Jesus Alvarez
  Robles, Francisco Javier Alvarez Rodriguez, and Edgard
  Benitez-Guerrero, editors.
Description: Hershey, Pa. : Engineering Science Reference, [2019]
Identifiers: LCCN 2018055857| ISBN 9781522585398 (hardcover) | ISBN
  9781522585404 (softcover) | ISBN 9781522585411 (ebook)
Subjects: LCSH: Blind, Apparatus for the--Technological innovations. | User
  interfaces (Computer systems) | Computers and people with disabilities. |
  Application software--Development.
Classification: LCC HV1664.P7 U84 2019 | DDC 005.1087/1--dc23 LC record available at https://
lccn.loc.gov/2018055857

This book is published in the IGI Global book series Advances in Systems Analysis, Software
Engineering, and High Performance Computing (ASASEHPC) (ISSN: 2327-3453; eISSN: 2327-
3461)

British Cataloguing in Publication Data
A Cataloguing in Publication record for this book is available from the British Library.

For electronic access to this publication, please contact: eresources@igi-global.com.

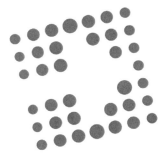

Advances in Systems Analysis, Software Engineering, and High Performance Computing (ASASEHPC) Book Series

ISSN:2327-3453
EISSN:2327-3461

Editor-in-Chief: Vijayan Sugumaran, Oakland University, USA

MISSION

The theory and practice of computing applications and distributed systems has emerged as one of the key areas of research driving innovations in business, engineering, and science. The fields of software engineering, systems analysis, and high performance computing offer a wide range of applications and solutions in solving computational problems for any modern organization.

The **Advances in Systems Analysis, Software Engineering, and High Performance Computing (ASASEHPC) Book Series** brings together research in the areas of distributed computing, systems and software engineering, high performance computing, and service science. This collection of publications is useful for academics, researchers, and practitioners seeking the latest practices and knowledge in this field.

COVERAGE

- Parallel Architectures
- Software Engineering
- Performance Modelling
- Metadata and Semantic Web
- Network Management
- Distributed Cloud Computing
- Computer System Analysis
- Virtual Data Systems
- Human-Computer Interaction
- Computer Graphics

IGI Global is currently accepting manuscripts for publication within this series. To submit a proposal for a volume in this series, please contact our Acquisition Editors at Acquisitions@igi-global.com or visit: http://www.igi-global.com/publish/.

Titles in this Series

For a list of additional titles in this series, please visit:
https://www.igi-global.com/book-series/advances-systems-analysis-software-engineering/73689

Interdisciplinary Approaches to Information Systems and Software Engineering
Alok Bhushan Mukherjee (North-Eastern Hill University Shillong, India) and Akhouri
Pramod Krishna (Birla Institute of Technology Mesra, India)
Engineering Science Reference • ©2019 • 299pp • H/C (ISBN: 9781522577843) • US $215.00

Cyber-Physical Systems for Social Applications
Maya Dimitrova (Bulgarian Academy of Sciences, Bulgaria) and Hiroaki Wagatsuma (Kyushu
Institute of Technology, Japan)
Engineering Science Reference • ©2019 • 440pp • H/C (ISBN: 9781522578796) • US $265.00

Integrating the Internet of Things Into Software Engineering Practices
D. Jeya Mala (Thiagarajar College of Engineering, India)
Engineering Science Reference • ©2019 • 293pp • H/C (ISBN: 9781522577904) • US $215.00

Analyzing the Role of Risk Mitigation and Monitoring in Software Development
Rohit Kumar (Chandigarh University, India) Anjali Tayal (Infosys Technologies, India) and
Sargam Kapil (C-DAC, India)
Engineering Science Reference • ©2018 • 308pp • H/C (ISBN: 9781522560296) • US $225.00

Handbook of Research on Pattern Engineering System Development for Big Data Analytics
Vivek Tiwari (International Institute of Information Technology, India) Ramjeevan Singh
Thakur (Maulana Azad National Institute of Technology, India) Basant Tiwari (Hawassa
University, Ethiopia) and Shailendra Gupta (AISECT University, India)
Engineering Science Reference • ©2018 • 396pp • H/C (ISBN: 9781522538707) • US $320.00

Incorporating Nature-Inspired Paradigms in Computational Applications
Mehdi Khosrow-Pour, D.B.A. (Information Resources Management Association, USA)
Engineering Science Reference • ©2018 • 385pp • H/C (ISBN: 9781522550204) • US $195.00

For an entire list of titles in this series, please visit:
https://www.igi-global.com/book-series/advances-systems-analysis-software-engineering/73689

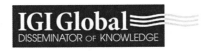

701 East Chocolate Avenue, Hershey, PA 17033, USA
Tel: 717-533-8845 x100 • Fax: 717-533-8661
E-Mail: cust@igi-global.com • www.igi-global.com

Editorial Advisory Board

Table of Contents

Section 2
Support Systems for the Blind and Visually Impaired

Foreword

According to the World Health Organization (2018), about 15% of the world population has some type of disability. In addition, estimates that there are 1300 million people with visual impairment in the world, of whom 36 million are diagnosed with blindness and 217 million people with moderate or severe visual impairment. It is also estimated that the number of children under 15 with visual disabilities amounts to 19 million.

In addition, this population faces great challenges for access to health, education and therefore to sources of quality employment. Some of these challenges are: prohibitive costs, physical barriers, limited availability of services, knowledge and management skills and interaction by the people responsible for education and health are inadequate, among others.

According to the World Report on Disability, the WHO (2018) warns that "People with disabilities are disadvantaged in terms of educational attainment and labor market outcomes," so that this generates clear sources of discrimination and inequality of opportunities. In the social and economic sphere, this may in some way be a cause of poverty and marginalization.

On the other hand, applied research and the development of technological solutions aimed at supporting populations with disabilities have had a greater boom at the academic level and in some companies, this is no exception. This is shown in this book *User-Centered Software Development for the Blind and Visually Impaired: Emerging Research and Opportunities*, which presents a series of relevant works for researchers and developers of technologies aimed at people with visual disabilities.

The authors address several issues from the design phases and inclusive strategies in software development and in particular of apps, to issues of user-centered design applied to the creation of learning resources. Various user experience evaluation techniques are adapted to the realities and needs of users with visual impairment, including HED / UT.

Chapter 1 presents a series of guides for the development of apps for support in orientation to people with visual disabilities in public transport. Chapter 2 develops inclusive design techniques, linking the paradigms of user-centered design and universal design for learning, in order to create educational strategies for people with visual disabilities. Chapter 3 presents a modification to the Hedonic utility scale as a method for measuring user experience in people with visual impairment.

Chapter 4 presents a technological solution based on mobile platforms for blind people, called as an audio-based mobile assistant for reading texts. Chapter 5 provides a set of factors to be considered when developing learning objects for people with visual disabilities, expanding these factors to consider the opinion of the user as well as the expert in the material of the learning object.

Chapter 6 presents the use of the "Team Software Process" methodology for the creation of a mobile application for people with visual disabilities in support of memory and learning about the city of Aguascalientes, Mexico, as a support for inclusion of this population in society. Chapter 7 presents the experience, based on qualitative research, on the use and adaptation of "logic blocks" as a manual support technology oriented towards inclusive pedagogical practices.

Chapter 8 presents the experience of designing applications to support the learning of Braille for people with visual disabilities. The authors are based on ISO15288:2015 standards and on adapted methods for the measurement of usability and user experience, used in blind people.

Finally, Chapter 9 proposes the use of artificial neural networks, an artificial intelligence technique, so that color blind people can learn the colors and can distinguish well when using Ishihara plates as input and recolor the image increasing its brightness.

In summary, the book *User-Centered Software Development for the Blind and Visually Impaired: Emerging Research and Opportunities* presents a series of high-value works that will serve as a reference and basis for future research, which I am sure will leave a great experience for its readers. Enjoy it and take advantage.

Mario Chacón Rivas
Tecnológico de Costa Rica, Costa Rica

Mario Chacón Rivas *is a Professor at the Costa Rican Institute of Technology (ITCR), Campus of Cartago. He holds a Ph.D. in Computer Science. He has published research papers in several international conferences in the topics of E-learning, learning objects, collaborative systems, databases, among others. His research interests are Information Technology, relational databases, virtualization, LMS, software engineering process for e-learning and collaborative systems. He is currently researcher of the INCLUTEC (inclusive technologies) and professor of the Costa Rican Institute of Technology (ITCR).*

REFERENCES

WHO. (2018, October 11). *Organización Mundial de la Salud*. Retrieved from https://www.who.int/es/news-room/fact-sheets/detail/blindness-and-visual-impairment

Preface

In this book we focus on the topic of User-Centered Software Development; specifically, in the development, implementation and analysis of software for blind and visually impaired.

The subject of the book, in general, is very important. In the last 10 years the development of software systems for blind people has been increasing; however, there are many cases in which the software has not been entirely useful for target users due to various factors, such as:

- Test performed by people with normal vision.
- Null evaluation tests.
- Assumption of reaction by the end user.
- Not taken into account users' opinions.

In several projects the target users do not participate in the evaluation tests of the software, for this reason we decided to prepare this book, to make known not only the importance but to show why it is important to take into account the blind or visual impaired user during the entire process development.

Information and communication technologies have advanced significantly in response to the needs of society in all areas: health, education, recreation, government, etc. In an increasingly globalized world, however, to date has not been achieved people with physical disabilities, cognitive disabilities, for example. This situation generates a line of work.

This material aims to show examples of how information and communication technologies can support in achieving these objectives of inclusion in the development of a fairer and more equitable society in the access to diverse applications and diverse utilities such as supporting the mobility of blind users, learning for the braille system on mobile devices, to name a few.

This work is aimed at specialists in the use and development of information and communication technologies interested in the topics of digital inclusion and reduction of the digital divide.

Although all the cases presented in this book are related to blind or visually impaired people, much of this material can serve as a conceptual and technical basis for other types of disabilities. In other words, those interested in developing technology for different disabilities could adapt the development methods presented, as well as the tools that evaluate usability and user experience.

We believe that the content of the book is a very useful tool not only for technologists but also specialists from other disciplines interested in this subject that allows generating new ideas and discussions around technology and disability (not only blind or visually impaired).

This book has been organized in three sections, to facilitate its reading and understanding of the contents: Section 1 – "Guides, Methods, and Strategies," considering the processes and different elements that allow developing inclusive technologies for blind and visually impaired people. Section 2 – "Support Systems for the Blind and Visually Impaired." Developed systems that allow to review and guarantee their use and Section 3 – "Extra." Additional cases related to the exposed topic.

Following is a brief overview of the chapters presented.

Chapter 1: Design for Blind Users – Guidelines for Developing Mobile Apps for Supporting Navigation of Blind People on Public Transports

This chapter covers the guidelines developers should follow when we create mobile applications to support visually impaired people in their use of public transports. In order to identify the best practices in the development of these apps, one should focus on the particularities, limitations and concerns of visually impaired people regarding their mobility, orientation and navigation on public transports. It's equally important to understand the existing technology and how these users interact with it, so that we can optimize the user experience, the accessibility and usability in future endeavors.

Chapter 2: Strategies and Technology Aids for Teaching Science to Blind and Visually Impaired Students

This chapter aims to provide a panorama of suitable teaching resources and strategies for science education of blind and visually impaired students. The authors will also present the foundations for designing inclusive learning materials based on the User-Centered Design and Universal Design for Learning (UDL) frameworks, using as example the development of technology-based tactile three-dimensional prototypes for teaching biology.

Chapter 3: Factors Determining Learning Objects Quality for People With Visual Impairment Integrating a Service Approach

This chapter has the objective of present which are the main factors that must be considered when we develop Learning Objects for people with visual impairment. The instruments for determine Learning Objects quality usually only consider the area expert perspective, without considering the user opinion. For the above, it is proposed to integrate aspects of service theory in the quality determination, in order to generate Learning Objects that also provide greater satisfaction of use to the student.

Chapter 4: Logic Blocks – Manual Assistive Technology for Visually Impaired Students

This chapter presents perceptions resulting from a piece of a continuing education course developed in conjunction with Basic Education teachers whose goal was to adapt and analyze the use of the Logic Blocks as a manual assistive technology, aiming inclusive pedagogical practices in the work performed in regular classes intended for visually impaired people's enrollment. It is about a qualitative research, outlined as research- formation.

Chapter 5: Hedonic Utility Scale (HED/UT) Modified as a User Experience Evaluation Method of Performing Talkback Tutorial for Blind People

In this chapter it is proposed to adapt the HED/UT Scale method for its application with blind users using the Google TalkBack tutorial as a case study. Based on Nielsen's Heuristics, five blind users rated the tutorial after completing each of its five tasks. To ensure inclusiveness in the adaptation of the method, this could be answered verbally and with the use of cards written in Braille, while, for questions of practicality in the evaluation, the number of items was reduced as well as changed the way of scoring (scale and equations) with respect to the original HED/UT. The results show that the Talkback tutorial is generally well accepted and well rated by users in both dimensions (hedonic and utility).

Chapter 6: Application Mobile Design for Blind People – History Memorama

The Team Software Process (TSP) is a methodology focused on software development on gears, which at the end of the construction ensures product quality (Humphrey,

2000). This quality must be considered for people with disabilities as it is visual impairment. This article focuses on using the TSP for the construction of an application for people with visual disabilities, resulting in a quality product that will help in the memory.

Chapter 7: Braille System Using an UX Evaluation Methodology Focused on the Use of Methods for Blind Users

In this chapter, we focus on making use of some tools that exist within the area of Software Engineering (SE) and user experience (UX) with the aim of developing an interactive software system (ISS). It is expected that this ISS will support people with visual disabilities to learn Braille. To develop the ISS, we use modified usability and UX evaluation methods for blind people. Based on the results, it is observed that the ISS complies with most of the UX factors, such as ease of use, accessibility and utility, so we expect the ISS to be usable for blind people

Chapter 8: Use of Audio-Based Mobile Assistant for Reading Texts as Support for Blind Users

In this chapter, we propose a technological solution based on the mobile platforms for the blind to perform tasks in the place and time necessary without more resources than a Smartphone.

Chapter 9: Real-Time Recoloring Ishihara Plates Using Artificial Neural Networks for Helping Colorblind People

In this chapter is proposed the use of artificial neural networks an artificial intelligence technique for learning the colors that colorblind people cannot distinguish well by using as input data the Ishihara plates and recoloring the image by increasing its bright. Results are tested with a real colorblind person, that successfully pass the Ishihara test.

In general, it can be indicated that this is an unpublished material that reflects the experiences of different research groups, considering from technology already implemented, as well as development and instrumentation strategies for new technologies. We believe that these chapters are a sample of many other works that are currently being developed but that have the wisdom to compile a common theme.

Acknowledgment

To the authors for their commitment since without their participation this book would not have been possible. To the reviewers for their time and commitment to deliver on time and form the requests by the editors. To the visually impaired people in general who were involved in each of the projects mentioned in the book.

Thank you all for making this project possible, with the purpose of publicizing the research and projects that are being carried out to support blind or low vision people in the field of Computer Science.

Section 1
Guides, Methods, and Strategies

Chapter 1
Designing for Blind Users:
Guidelines for Developing Mobile Apps for Supporting Navigation of Blind People on Public Transports

Ana Cristina Antunes
Polytechnic Institute of Lisbon, Portugal

Camila Silva
IPAM, Portugal

ABSTRACT

This chapter covers the guidelines developers should follow when creating mobile applications to support visually impaired people in their use of public transports. Technology has evolved in a remarkable fashion, mobile applications being the perfect example of a resource that has been solving problems for a vast array of users, including visually impaired people. These apps hold tremendous potential seeing as they present an accessible, multi-functioned, and cost-effective solution to the mobility issues impacting visually impaired people. In order to identify the best practices in the development of these apps, one should focus on the particularities, limitations, and concerns of visually impaired people regarding their mobility, orientation, and navigation on public transports. It's equally important to understand the existing technology and how these users interact with it, so that we can optimize the user experience, the accessibility, and usability in future endeavors.

DOI: 10.4018/978-1-5225-8539-8.ch001

INTRODUCTION

In the last decades, technology has advanced at an astonishing pace. Technological progress has brought changes in many contexts, from the workplace to the classroom and even to daily life. The impact of these technological advances has been so pervasive that has extended to many different types of users, such as people who are visually impaired. Demographic trends reveal that this specific type of users, including those who are blind, are a wide audience of users and that their number will grow in the next years.

According to the latest information provided by the World Health Organization (WHO, 2018), based on the study of Bourne et al. (2017), there are approximately 253 million people with vision impairment, including 36 million who are blind. Visual impairment is defined in the International Statistical Classification of Diseases - ICT (2018), as deficits in the ability of the person to perform vision-related activities of daily living. Visual impairment ranges from moderate and severe vision impairment, both grouped under the term "low vision", to blindness. Blindness can be defined as having visual acuity less than 3/60 in the better eye (ICT, 2018).

Recent and prospective studies reveal that the number of visually impaired people has increased in the last years and is expected to increase. According to the data provided by Bourne et al. (2017), from 1990 until 2017, the number of blind people and people with moderate and severe visual impairment has increased, respectively by 17,6% and 35,4%. Furthermore, it is estimated that the number of blind people in the world will largely increase in the next decades, due both to population growth and aging. Indeed, WHO (2017) estimates that by 2050 there could be 115 million people who are blind.

Besides demographics, another relevant issue to consider regarding the visually impaired adults is their reported poorer or declining health in comparison to sighted adults (e.g,, Capella-McDonnall, 2007), a disparity in part caused by less physical activity in the visually impaired population due to real and perceived barriers, including walking alone (e.g., Rimmer & Braddock, 2002). Individuals with visual impairments face several difficulties in what concerns independent mobility, such as traveling and navigating in public spaces or using public transports, which considerably deprive them of a typical professional and social functioning (Tuttle & Tuttle, 2004), shaping their social inclusion and quality of life (Lubin & Deka, 2012; Long et al., 2016). Their social and professional exclusion, in turn, reinforces their experiences of disablement (e.g., Wong, 2018). Therefore, it is critical to examine and address the assistive technologies available for these users, especially the ongoing advances in information technology (IT) that are increasing the scope for IT-based mobile assistive technologies for mobility and navigation that, as Hakobyan et al. (2013) defend, can increase the independence, safety, and improve the overall quality of life of the visually impaired.

Since individuals with different degrees of visual impairment present diverse mobility and navigation concerns and constraints, in this chapter the focus will be on the distinct experiences, abilities, and limitations of blind people. One of the streams of research concerning IT-based assistive technologies for visually-impaired people has been on mobile phones equipped with specific mobile applications (apps) and other handheld devices accessible via haptic (touch) and audio sensory channels. The current domain of IT-based assistive technologies for visually-impaired people is broad, as well as the range of support that these technologies can provide. In this chapter and based on an extensive literature review, the focus is on the guidelines for developing apps to support blind users' mobility, orientation, and navigation in public transports.

CHARACTERISTICS AND LIMITATIONS OF BLIND PEOPLE

It is fundamental to consider that visually impaired people present several specificities, constraints, and limitations as users, and these must be attended to and considered when designing any type of assistive technologies for them.

At a cultural level, and specifically focusing on blind users, Tuunanen (2003) and Hebler, Tuunanen and Peffers (2007) refer that these users are widely dispersed, since they come from very diverse cultures and places and, in certain cases, have their own group culture, so web and mobile designers may not intuitively understand their needs and preferences (e.g., Overby, Woodruff, & Gardial, 2005). They also have a differential access to assistive technologies, due to social and economic factors.

At a biological level, the brain has the neuroplasticity required to reconnect and distribute resources from one sense to another. For example, in blind people the resources that would usually be allocated to their vision may migrate to their touch and hearing areas. According to Troancã et al. (2015) for them to benefit from their unique aptitudes and to obtain the best results, their learning processes should mainly focus on haptic and sound stimuli.

Carroll (1961), who studied the specificities of visually impaired people, concluded that the senses are often used to perceive the surrounding world. Even though his conclusions aren't yet unanimous, there's an ongoing scientific discussion on how visually impaired people develop their remaining senses to compensate for their lack of sight. This compensatory dynamic can impact how blind people perceive and orientate themselves in the surrounding world.

Cattaneo and Vecchi (2011) have presented three different theories on sensory compensation in blindness. The first one claims that no sense is dependent on any other for efficiency or development. Another theory defends that sight is essential for the development and efficiency of the remaining senses, meaning that a blind person will also experience limitations on their other senses. The last theory presented by these authors claims that the senses are significantly optimized when compensating for the absence of one sense. Nevertheless, blind people must rely on their remaining senses to overcome their daily challenges, which inadvertently makes them more practiced and attuned.

Merabet and Pascual-Leone (2010) refer to Braille readers as has having a more developed sense of touch, and this might be related to the demands of learning Braille. Röder and Rösler (2003) concluded that blind people are more skilled in terms of tactile acuity, compared to people with sight, due to their practice and intensive use of their sense of touch. These authors state that the brain plasticity in blind people is triggered by the learning process and by motor and perceptual training.

Purves et al. (2004) explain the implications and the potential of our brain to adapt and respond to certain needs. According to them, the brain has the ability and flexibility needed to learn new skills, establish new memories and deal with injuries throughout life.

The capacity for memorization relates to the ideas previously presented about neurologic flexibility and plasticity as both can be considered tools that facilitate, optimize and support perceptive and sensorial activities for these individuals. Harrar et al. (2018) claim that memory helps blind people with perceiving the surrounding environment. These authors defend that in order to memorize anything in a precise manner, one should combine sensations, senses, and emotional stimuli. They approach the concept of sensorial memory, used as a reference point, when applied to spatial recognition.

ISSUES REGARDING MOBILITY, NAVIGATION AND ORIENTATION OF BLIND PEOPLE

As Giudice and Legge (2008) indicate, sometimes the navigational components of orientation and mobility are used interchangeably in the literature. Yet, their notions point to different properties of human locomotion and involve different capabilities of exploration of the environment (Cuturi et al., 2016). Orientation refers to the ability to recognize the spatial properties of the environment and to establish one's position in relation to the environment (Hill & Ponder, 1976) when navigating from point A to point B. Orientation involves body, objects and space conscience, as well as efficient perceptive moving behavior and the adequate use of these concepts (Novi, 1998).

On the other hand, mobility can be defined as the ability to physically move from one place to another (Koutny & Miesenberger, 2014), that is, to move safely, orderly and efficiently through the environment unaccompanied (for instance, travel alone to a hospital using a public transport) and independently (Novi, 1998). Good mobility relates to efficient locomotion and orientation to accurate wayfinding behavior (Giudice & Legge, 2008) and involves detecting, avoiding or negotiating obstacles and hazards, establishing and maintaining the desired course, and recovery from unintended or unexpected changes in direction (e.g,, Bradley & Dunlop, 2008; Giudice & Legge, 2008). Both orientation and mobility allow good navigation, that is, the purposeful process involved in traveling from one place to another, using mobility skills, and orientation in the environment attending the desired course (Bradley & Dunlop, 2008).

Orientation and mobility in humans rely heavily on sight. Indeed, while navigating, sighted individuals rely on multisensory information, integrating auditory and mobility cues with vision (e.g., Gori et al., 2017). This multisensory integration allows them to update their body position in the space and orientate themselves within a given environment (e.g., Loomis et al., 1993). Yet, the visual experience plays a critical role in shaping space perception and representation, since vision is the major source of spatial information and dominates spatial perception over other sensory modalities (e.g., Cuturi et al., 2016; Eimer, 2004). Our senses are inextricably linked, and our perception of visual, auditory or tactile events can be dramatically altered by information from other senses (Eimer, 2004) or their lacking. Considering this and attending to vision's major role in space perception, in the absence of vision, such as occurs in blindness, navigation and mobility capabilities may result compromised (e.g., Gori et al., 2017). Indeed, blind individuals don't have access to the visual experience, and therefore lack this fundamental sensory signal for orientation, mobility, and navigation.

According to Golledge et al. (1996), blind people explore cognitive techniques for memorization for better spatial orientation and use them to map their surrounding environment as well as the routes they plan on taking. In this sense, a visually impaired traveler has to establish relations between different reference points, sensations, objects, movement or memorized directions.

Although compensatory mechanisms can be adopted to improve blind people's spatial and navigation capabilities (e.g., Gori et al., 2017), some studies suggest an impaired performance in blind individuals in inferential navigation (e.g., Rieser, Guth, & Hill, 1986; Seemungal et al., 2007). According to Nakamura (1997), early blind individuals also show a slower walking speed, a more cautious posture, a shorter stride length and a longer duration of stance, when compared with late blind and sighted individuals. Yet, Cuturi et al. (2016) suggest some caution while comparing sighted and blind individuals since the literature still presents some inconsistent results.

However, when we consider that even simple travel activities to known places, such as a bus journey across a city to go to work or to visit a relative by bus, metro or railway, generates a long list of travel subtasks (Harper & Green, 2000), and that visually impaired individuals have limited transportation options (e.g., Wong, 2018), we understand that orientation and mobility in urban areas can be a challenging and emotionally stressful task for the blind. Additionally, most existing urban environments were not designed with accessibility in mind and consequently many visually impaired people experience severe difficulties in traveling even short distances in these public spaces (Hersch & Johnson, 2008). In this context, the development of travel aids that facilitate mobility and independent travel by blind people is an important application area for assistive technology (Hersch & Johnson, 2008).

Traveling to unknown destinations and navigating in unfamiliar outdoor environments can even be more challenging, since blind people lack much of the information needed for planning detours around obstacles and hazards, and have little information about distant landmarks, heading and self-velocity (Loomis, Golledge, & Klatzky, 2001). Attending to this, it is not surprising that the more severe a visual impairment, the more likely a person is to experience a decline in mobility (Aartolahti et al., 2013; Salive et al., 1994).

BLIND PEOPLE PLANNING AND EXPERIENCE OF TRAVELLING USING PUBLIC TRANSPORTS

To understand how blind people use mobile IT assistive technology when they travel by using public transports and the main principles and guidelines for designing this technology, one must first comprehend their routines, habits, needs, and difficulties or problems related to traveling.

According to Sánchez and Sáenz (2006), prior to any travel, the blind must obtain three levels of knowledge, to be able to travel in a safe, independent way: (1) Conceptual, that is, to understand basic and generic concepts regarding bus, subway or train network in any city of the world. Once these concepts are learned, the user can proceed to the next level; (2) Knowledge, this involves knowing specific information of a particular bus or subway network, such as the bus stop or station name, the surroundings, the location, and lines names that identify a route or path (transfer and local); and (3) Articulation, that is, to use these different concepts and knowledge learned by the user for an efficient use of the bus, train or subway network. This includes planning of the travel, as well as estimation and cost.

Planning seems to be a relevant issue, especially when traveling to unknown places. Kane et al. (2009) describe how blind people use information for planning trips to unknown places before leaving home. When visiting a place for the first time, it is frequent for blind people to try to pull several pieces of information together, to plan their journey. This preparation includes looking up directions, checking bus schedules, and calling ahead to ask about accessibility features. In a qualitative research with 10 blind people, Silva (2017) found that planning is also usually done and considered as useful when traveling to already known places. Available transports and schedules, the need to exchange line or transport, streets or places prohibited by construction works, public road configuration, and travel simulations are attended to in this planning.

Based on the results obtained from the interviews to 13 blind or deaf-blind people, Azenkot et al. (2011) suggest that the main challenges experienced by blind people, when using a bus to travel, were locating a stop, knowing where they are during the travel and disembarking at the correct bus stop. On the other hand, Minifie and Cody (2009) refer as main problems finding the right bus, finding the bus door and staying independent. Besides the problems stated, when travelling to new or unfamiliar places, blind people are also preoccupied with station or bus stop accessibility, physical obstacles in their way, identification of railway, bus or subway lines and destinations, as well as the possibility and/or potential problems of circulating with a guide dog (Silva, 2017).

Prior to the availability and dissemination of mobile technology, blind people relied on bus drivers or other travelers to obtain the necessary information during the travel. This is well expressed in the routines of public transportation use identified by Azenkot et al. (2011). According to their study, when blind participants intended to use a bus and reached a stop's identifying intersection, they would search for a stop pole or shelter, a group of people waiting at the stop, or ask for directions to a nearby pedestrian. Knowing which landmarks were at the stop and where they were located within the street was helpful. When a bus arrived at a stop, participants asked the driver or other riders for its route. When multiple buses reached a stop at the same time they felt stressed. Once in the desired bus, participants relied on the bus driver to know when to disembark the bus on unfamiliar routes.

Mobile devices and mobile applications (apps) have the potential to change this landscape and reshape everyday mobilities for blind individuals, introducing new patterns in travel routines. Connected mobile devices have globally evolved into extremely effective tools that support travelers, since mobile devices and apps provide comprehensive information services for travel planning, travel facilitation, and travel communication (Wang & Xiang, 2012). Today, when blind people travel alone and independently, they often make use of orientation and mobility devices and tools (e.g., long canes and dog guides) but can also use orientation and navigation technology (e.g., global positioning systems, such as GPS, or navigational apps) (Kaiser, Cmar, Rosen & Anderson, 2018).

Mobile devices and navigational apps have shifted the power over access to real-time information, for instance allowing a blind person to obtain updated GPS information, spatial information about the immediate surroundings, or the direction that the user is walking in, the distance to street crossings, or even public transit arrival times (Wong, 2018). Apps can also be of use in situations where the capability, coupling, and authority constraints associated with using public transportation are too high (Wong, 2018). As examples, when blind people get lost while traveling, are late for an appointment, miss a bus or train, live in a rural area where public transports are fewer or the journey involves the coordination and use of too many public transports, they can use an app to call for a ride-hailing service such as Uber.

In spite of these and other advantages, the most commonly used mobility devices by blind people are still the long cane and the guide dog (Gori et al., 2016; Hersh, 2018a, 2018b), instead of other available alternatives. Hersh (2018a) presents several reasons for the low use of other mobility devices, that range from high costs, weight, lack of easily available, limited benefits compared to the long cane, difficulties involved in learning how to use these devices, unattractive and obtrusive appearance to lack of information regarding what is available. In the next section, the authors briefly examine IT-based assistive technologies to support orientation and navigation of visually-impaired people. The focus will be placed on the role of apps as an assistive technology that supports the mobility and navigation of blind users while discussing how these apps can surpass the problems raised by Hersh (2018a).

IT-BASED ASSISTIVE TECHNOLOGIES FOR THE BLIND

Recently, there has been a rise of interest in the development of technological solutions for assisting the visually impaired people (Cuturi et al., 2016) in their everyday activities. As a result, several platforms and systems have emerged in the last years (e.g., Brito et al., 2018).

Focusing on orientation and navigation for blind people, Lin, Lee, and Chiang (2017) provide a brief categorization and description of the existing devices, considering three categories: electronic travel aids, electronic orientation aids, and position locator devices.

Electronic travel aids, or ETAs, are general assisting devices that help visually impaired people avoid obstacles. Their sensory inputs may come from a depth camera, a general camera, radio frequency identification (RFID), an ultrasonic sensor, or an infrared sensor (e.g., Lin, Lee & Chiang, 2017).

Electronic orientation aids, or EOAs, are designed to aid visually impaired people in finding their way in a new and unknown environment (e.g., Lin, Lee & Chiang, 2017). EOAs generally require much environmental information to examine the surroundings. To provide a guiding service that involves the recognition of possible obstacles, it is usual for these systems to combine a camera with multiple sensors (e.g., Hoang et al., 2017).

Position locator devices, or PLDs, are devices used to determine the precise position of its holder, encompassing global positioning system (GPS) and geographic information system (GIS) technologies (e.g., Adagale & Mahajan, 2015; Bahadur & Tripathi, 2016). GPS and GIS-based guiding systems for blind people can find the current location and guide the blind user from the present location to the destination and give an alert at the arrival to the destination area (Lin, Lee & Chiang, 2017).

Despite all the investment that has been made, well expressed in the variety of existing technological solutions available for the visually impaired, the existing technologies still present downsides and limitations (e.g., Koutny & Miesenberger, 2014; Long et al., 2016; Lin, Lee & Chiang, 2017). For instance, position locator devices usually rely on GPS for positioning, but this technology cannot guarantee an accurate precision or accuracy in general, cannot help the blind users avoiding the obstacles in front of them and can fail in routes between high buildings (e.g., Brito et al., 2018; Koutny & Miesenberger, 2014; Lin, Lee & Chiang, 2017).

It has been suggested that these technological devices developed to support the visually impaired should present an integrated, multifunctional, transparent and extensive solution (Hersh, 2018a) to their orientation and mobility problems. But to date, no single technological device has succeeded in this.

As already stated, the cane and the guide dog are still the most used auxiliaries for navigation by visually impaired people (Gori et al., 2016; Hersh, 2018a, 2018b). But more recently, mobile devices have become more accessible (Dobosz, 2016) and mobile applications (apps) have been gaining ground and acceptance from researchers, designers, and blind users as assistive technologies. Indeed, in the study of Silva (2017), the blind participants referred that they used several navigational apps, such as AriadneGPS, Moovit, Google Maps, and ViaOpta Nav, when they use public transports.

Apps seem to be particularly promising as an assistive technology for visually impaired individuals (Long et al., 2016), including the blind. Their main advantages are their portability, cost-effectiveness, easy access to information everywhere and anytime, and ease of use (Griffin-Shirley et al., 2017). Navigational apps, among other devices, have also shifted the power over access in real-time information from everyone else back to the blind (Wong, 2018), empowering these users.

Nowadays, apps cannot provide complete and integrated solutions to assist mobility and orientation of blind users, given their limited ability to enhance the navigational capacities of blind people. But apps can be joined with well-established assistive technologies, such as canes, to facilitate daily travel or access to transportation (Wong, 2018).

Given their recency and notwithstanding their potential benefits for blind people, the use of apps for people with visual impairments is still scarcely researched (e.g., Griffin-Shirley et al., 2017; Wong, 2018). In a recent study that involved 259 participants with visual impairments, Griffin-Shirley et al. (2017) found that they were globally satisfied with apps and considered them as useful and accessible. Although, they would like to see improvements made to existing apps and suggest the development of useful new apps to people with visual impairments. This is a relevant issue, also raised by Sierra and de Togores (2012), who suggest that apps should be developed for the visually impaired or even specifically for the blind, instead of being designed for sighted users and include accessibility features. When designing an app for the blind, there is, according to Sierra and de Togores (2012), a considerable improvement in usability and, ultimately, a better user experience. Conception and development of an app specifically for a target with disabilities implies not only attending to accessibility but also following specific principles and guidelines for better app design. Good design does not guarantee the success of a new device, but paying attention to design principles and guidelines can lead to better device design, meaning that the app is more likely to be used by a significant number of people (Hersh, 2018a).

FROM ACCESSIBILITY TO SPECIFIC GUIDELINES FOR THE DEVELOPMENT OF APPS TO SUPPORT ORIENTATION AND MOBILITY OF BLIND USERS IN PUBLIC TRANSPORTS

When designing mobile applications for people with disabilities, designers must attend to accessibility (e.g., Rodriguez-Sanchez & Martinez-Romo, 2017; Sierra & de Togores, 2012). The Web Accessibility Initiative (WAI), an organization affiliated with the World Wide Web Consortium (W3C), promotes and develops accessibility standard guidelines. Among these, WAI (2018) suggests the Mobile Web Accessibility Guideline (MWAG) as a set of mobile accessibility guidelines, based on the Web Content Accessibility Guidelines (WCAG) 2.0, for addressing accessibility issues in mobile webpages and mobile applications. These include four guidelines: the web content must be perceivable, operable, understandable, and robust.

To address accessible mobile application design, Park, Goh and So (2015) interviewed people with visual impairment to understand their user experiences when using smartphones and mobile applications. They employed a heuristic walkthrough method to develop a set of accessibility guidelines specifically for people with visual impairment. These mobile application accessibility guidelines are presented in Table 1.

The main goal of these accessibility standards and guidelines is to help design apps that any person with visual impairment can use. Notwithstanding its importance and interest, one must also observe that this target presents a huge variation regarding sight: people with moderate visual impairments and people with low vision have differences between them; both groups are different and present different needs, specificities and limitations when compared with blind people. These differences must be attended to when designing mobile applications.

The remainder of this chapter describes several guidelines for designing apps that support orientation, mobility, and navigation of blind people in public transports.

Table 1. Mobile application accessibility guidelines for people with visual impairment

Guidelines	Guidelines description
Substitutive text	Provide a substitutive text to all user interface (UI) components.
Object with focus	Every object can get a focus and this focus is the most important concept to people with visual impairment. The focus acts as a computer mouse. It is a very natural concept to point everything using a mouse.
Logical focus flow	Provide a logical focus flow. People with visual impairment should receive information in a focused order. The focus sequence should be designed with consideration of information completeness.
Operating system accessibility support	Use accessibility functions and properties provided by the operating system of companies such as Apple and Google, because it is easy to provide compatibility with other assistive devices.
Press action support	Provide control with a press action. All controls should be handled with a press action.
Simple structure	Provide a simple structure and under 30 items at one page. When there are too many items on a page, people with visual impairment have trouble browsing. Simple structure helps focus configuration.
Substitutive action	Provide a substitutive button on overlapped action.
Notice function	Provide, as much as possible, various notice methods. Every information on screen should have more than two methods and exploit various sensory functions.
Consistent UI	Provide consistent placement for UI components. UI component placement should be consistent to increase learnability.

Source: (Park, Goh, & So, 2015)

Adopting a user-centric perspective and based on the existing literature, two sets of guidelines are presented: one set related to the planning of the travel and the other to the travel itself. Indeed, when traveling, planning the journey seems to be an aspect of the utmost importance for the blind (e.g., Kane et al., 2009; Sánchez & Sáenz, 2006), and influences their level of confidence before and during the travel. Attending to this, mobile applications should include functionalities related to travel planning. Table 2 presents the specific guidelines that should be considered when designing these functionalities.

Planning the Travel

According to the literature, one of the reasons for planning a trip, besides the efficient management of public transport, is the optimized access to information about the route (e.g., Chen et al., 2015; Kane et al., 2009 Sánchez & Oyarzún, 2008). The use of reference points along the journey facilitates and optimizes the recognition and guidance of the user in the space. These elements are included in the guideline "Availability of information", described in Table 2.

Azenkot et al. (2011) study reveal that independence, trust and safety are key values for the blind that rely on public transportation for everyday mobility. Safety emerged as a centrally important value in this context. This has clear implications for one of the guidelines included in Table 2, "Indicating the best itinerary or route". Providing several alternative routes or paths, with a clear indication of the fastest, most accessible, and safest itinerary increases autonomy, and safety for these users. But blind people prioritize safety over duration (Azenkot et al., 2011). Therefore, if there is a significant time difference between alternative routes, it should be the safest and not the fastest or shortest route to be suggested (e.g., Silva, 2017). For instance, with ViaOpta Nav, a navigation app developed by Novartis, waypoints can be added to improve the effectiveness of a calculated route.

These and the remaining guidelines for the design of mobile applications that address the issue of planning the travel can be consulted in Table 2.

Attending to the information gathered by Silva (2017), the travel planning functionality is often used by blind users in the exploration of unknown locations. Therefore, it is important that apps that assist blind users in mobility, orientation and navigation in public transports allow prior recognition of the space, including the anticipation of obstacles and even a travel simulation, to allow the blind user build a mental map of the route.

Table 2. Mobile application guidelines for planning the travel

Guidelines	Guidelines description
Availability of information	Provide relevant and updated information on schedules, stop locations, ticket price, reference points, and estimated travel duration. Detailed information is important but not always better. Therefore, the available information should provide useful content of a proper length.
Travel simulation	Include a description of the travel until the destination. Itinerary descriptions are the best way to guide users. Consider the possibility of the blind user consult a map or explore the route.
Anticipating obstacles	Assist the blind user on obstacles anticipation in their route, including construction works. Include alerts with information regarding the existence and localization of bicycle paths.
Indicating the best itinerary or route	Provide several alternative routes or paths, with a clear indication of the most accessible and safest itinerary.
Previous buying of tickets	All users must be able to acquire their tickets or transportation titles in an accessible and equitable manner. Sometimes, blind people have problems in acquiring the tickets at the ticket office. The app should provide previous ticket buying as a functionality.
Avoid app hierarchy	Avoid adding the app hierarchy. Search results should be displayed directly on the same page instead of jumping to another.

Source: (Chen et al., 2015; Kane et al., 2009; Sánchez & Oyarzún, 2008; Silva, 2017)

Using Public Transports

Several content guidelines are related to the synchronization and reliability of the information that is shared with the user, as can be seen in Table 3. The blind user must be able to access all the necessary information from the app, to manage his/her public transport travel with efficiency, independence, and safety, since they prefer to get information from the system than asking people around them (Azenkot et al., 2011).

It must be ensured that the blind user has access to useful information about the bus and the route at all stages of the journey (e.g., Brito et al., 2018; Lopes et al., 2012; Silva, 2017). When contextual information about the trip is scarce, orientation is very difficult for the blind, making it almost impossible for them to identify their position on the route with certainty (e.g., Azenkot et al., 2011) and to make the best and safest decisions about the travel. All the information that contextualizes the user on the location, on the identification of public transport, its schedule and the stops it makes during the trip is useful. For example, AriadneGPS offers blind users the possibility to know their position at any time and monitor it while walking. It also allows the possibility of exploring a map by using VoiceOver and to be informed about changes along the route or know street names.

Table 3. Mobile application guidelines to support public transportation use

Guidelines	Guidelines description
Availability of information regarding the arrival of public transport	Provide updated information on the time of waiting for the arrival of the public transport to the station/stop. Provide also an indication or alert on the coming of the public transport to the platform or stop, with a clear identification of the destination. Designers should keep in mind that detailed information is important but not always better. Therefore, there should be useful content of a proper length.
Availability of contextual spatial information	Provide contextual spatial information during the journey to increase control and independence on the blind user. Inform about the streets and important landmarks near each bus stop or station. Allow the user to access this information during the trip and, in case of a detour or the suspension of service, offer the blind user alternative services to complete the trip. Provide a previous and clear indication if is needed a transfer for another public transport or line.
Availability of information in real-time about the itinerary	Real-time information is essential since these users cannot use vision to know where they are. Provide real-time information on the estimated time of arrival or on other references points previously selected by the user. Provide a real-time indication of the stops name and distance to the next stop or station.
Availability of information regarding the arrival to the destination	Identifying when a bus, metro or metro arrive at the desired point of arrival is a major concern for blind users. Provide an alert on the arrival of the public transport to the desired destination.
Enabling the selection of directional instructions	Global directions and cardinal points (East, West, North, and South) are too abstract for the blind to understand. But there are several strategies that can be adopted for communicating directions, such as degrees, clock directions or proportional directions. Allow blind users to choose their preferred way of obtaining directions.
Providing guidance	Provide guidance to the nearest help point when the blind user gets lost.
Enabling dictation for selection of options	Enable the blind user with the possibility of dictating their selection from a list of options to reduce effort and time cost of selecting an item on the app. It also may be of use to ask for the previous instruction to be repeated or make a selection from a list.
Providing sequential instructions	Provide each information or instruction sequentially. Human beings do not deal well with an overload of information.
Enabling saving frequently used destinations or personal landmarks	To reduce effort, increase safety and provide a more personalized user experience, enable the blind user to save the most frequent destinations and the preferred landmarks.

Source: (Brito et al., 2018; Bujacz et al., 2008; Chen et al., 2015; Martins et al., 2016; Lopes et al., 2012; Sanchez & Oyarzún, 2008; Silva, 2017; Wayfindr, 2018)

In this chapter, the guidelines that refer to the availability of information are organized according to the main stages of a trip on public transport: the arrival of the transport, during the trip and the arrival at the destination. It is understood that to assist mobility and navigation in public transport the priority must be placed on sharing updated and real-time information (e.g., Silva, 2017). Moovit, an app that although is not specifically targeted for blind people is used by some of them for mobility (as can be seen in the study of Silva, 2017), provides information of real-time arrivals and alerts. Users can receive real-time arrival updates, which are taken directly from GPS devices positioned on buses and trains, as well as real-time alerts, such as emergency or unexpected disruptions, delays or traffic jams.

The amount and type of information provided should always be examined. It must be taken in account that an increased cognitive load, for instance from processing acoustical and/or tactile signals, might overwhelm the cognitive abilities of the blind user (Gori et al., 2016). As a result, both the user interface and function design should be simple, so it will not distract users (e.g., Chen et al., 2015). Besides being simple, the information presented to the blind users along the bus, train or metro route must be very concrete, and provided in a sequential basis (e.g., Brito et al., 2018), to avoid an overload of information that may confuse blind users. For instance, in the INCLUSO app developed by Brito et al. (2018), very concrete messages are provided to visually impaired people along the bus touring of the historic center of Viana do Castelo. These messages intend to locate the user as being near a bank or a garden, so he knows where to stop. It also provides information on the proximity of the crossings, so the user can leave the bus and safely cross the street.

Information on transfer stations between different bus and metro or train lines can also be of use.

It is also relevant to provide the possibility for people who are blind to obtain information on their physical/spacial surroundings, namely contextual information on streets, landmarks, and places of interest along the routes that are being navigated, such as museums or restaurants (e.g., Sanchez & Oyarzún, 2008). Describing the surrounding environment is one of the main functionalities of the app prototype presented by Dornhofer et al. (2014), which allows the user to explore the whole trip on the screen. This app also provides turn instruction by turn instruction and periodically gives an indication of the distance to the next crossing point. LocalEyes, developed by Behmer and Knox (2010), is a GPS-based application that intends to facilitate visually-impaired users' navigation and awareness of their environment. It allows them to explore information on surrounding points of interest, including restaurants, coffee-shops, etc.

Communicating the direction is fundamental for the orientation and navigation of the blind user. Yet, there are several possible strategies that can be adopted for this communication. Using cardinal points (East, West, North, and South) can be too abstract for the blind to understand (Chen et al., 2015), but there are many other alternatives. For instance, it can be used clock directions, degrees (e.g., turn at 90 degrees to your right), proportional directions (e.g., turn slightly to your right) or using the smartphones internal compass which will allow for more accurate angular directions (Wayfindr, 2018). Attending that blind users come from very diverse cultures and places (e.g., Hebler, Tuunanen, & Peffers, 2007; Tuunanen, 2003) and can have different experiences and knowledge regarding this matter, enabling them to select their preferred way of obtaining directional instructions can provide them a better user experience.

When a blind passenger gets lost in a given environment, such as a station, it is important to provide guidance on how to seek help as well as guide him/her to the nearest help point (e.g., Silva, 2017; Wayfindr, 2018). One of the guidelines included in Table 3 refers to the need of the designer include a functionality that can provide clear guidance in these cases.

Enabling saving of most frequent destinations reduces the effort required from the blind users (e.g., Wayfindr, 2018). Landmarks are also relevant for them during their navigation (e.g., Azenkot et al., 2011; Loomis, Golledge, & Klatzky, 2001) and enabling saving these landmarks reduces effort and allows to use them repeatedly for various purposes. For example, blind people might use the landmarks as a reassurance that they are on the right track, as a meeting point, etc. Moreover, allowing saving of personal landmarks with language that is more meaningful to each individual user is likely to provide a more personalized user experience (Wayfindr, 2018).

AriadneGPS provides the functionality of saving the favorite points and to be alerted, when the blind person approaches one of them, by using sound, vibration, or even voice, if is using VoiceOver.

CONCLUSION

It is widely recognized that blind people have difficulties moving and navigating independently in public transportation (e.g., Engelbrektsson et al., 2004; Martins et al., 2016; Sanchez & Oyarzún, 2008), especially in unfamiliar outdoor environments (Loomis, Golledge, & Klatzky, 2001). To overcome these obstacles, they make use of a vast array of tools to assist them in autonomous navigation and travel, from a walking stick for identifying obstacles and changes in the floor to a guide dog or to optical or IT-based assistive technologies. Within this context, mobile applications (apps) seem to be particularly promising as an assistive technology for orientation, mobility, and navigation of blind individuals because of their portability, cost-effectiveness, easy access to information, and ease of use (Griffin-Shirley et al., 2017). Apps designed to support the mobility of blind users in public transports can significantly influence their levels of safety, confidence, and independence (e.g., Azenkot et al., 2011; Silva, 2017), empowering these users. Since the integration of blind people into daily societal activities requires accessibility to all modes of transportation available in the city, in order to make independent travel to and from different points (Sanchez et al., 2013), apps that assist this user in this context can facilitate their autonomy and integration in society and improve their overall quality of life (e.g., Hakobyan et al., 2013; Lubin & Deka, 2012; Long et al., 2016).

Departing from a review the existing literature on the blind user and the field of mobile assistive technology for this user, this chapter highlights the role of apps as an assistive technology that supports the mobility and navigation of blind users in public transports. The focus of the chapter is on what the researchers and designers point as best practices, examining the main guidelines that must be followed in the development of apps to address these users' needs regarding mobility, orientation, and navigation in public transports.

Since the use of mobile technology for blind people is still scarcely researched (e.g., Griffin-Shirley et al., 2017; Wong, 2018), additional research is required in this field. In the future, researchers should investigate what other functionalities are needed in apps that support orientation, mobility, and navigation of blind people, as well as the main problems blind users face, in order to present, as Hersh (2018a) suggests, an integrated, multifunctional, and extensive solution for their mobility and orientation challenges and difficulties. This integrated solution may pose different accessibility issues that need to be addressed, as well as the need for additional guidelines.

The authors also agree with the suggestion of Long et al. (2016) regarding the need for further research on the best way to communicate visual cues to visually impaired people, bridging current accessibility gaps. Furthermore, since designers of these type of interfaces do not usually have visual impairments and have a limited understanding of blind user experiences with mobile devices and apps (Rodriguez-Sanchez & Martinez-Romo, 2017), there is a need of more research to understand how blind people use mobile technology, on their specificities and limits, and when and where they use it in articulation with other technological solutions.

Another stream of research could examine which factors promote these apps adoption and engagement. For instance, what built-in features are more relevant for blind users and influence app acceptance and adoption, or what are the main drivers of engagement when specifically considering apps that support orientation, mobility, and navigation of blind people.

REFERENCES

Aartolahti, E., Häkkinen, A., Lönnroos, E., Kautiainen, H., Sulkava, R., & Hartikainen, S. (2013). Relationship between functional vision and balance and mobility performance in community-dwelling older adults. *Aging Clinical and Experimental Research*, 25(5), 545–552. doi:10.100740520-013-0120-z PMID:24002802

Adagale, V., & Mahajan, S. (2015). Route guidance system for blind people using GPS and GSM. *International Journal of Electrical and Electronic Engineering & Telecommunications*, 4(2), 16–21.

AriadneG. P. S. (n.d.). Retrieved from http://www.ariadnegps.eu/

Azenkot, S., Prasain, S., Borning, A., Fortuna, E., Ladner, R. E., & Wobbrock, J. (2011). Enhancing independence and safety for blind and deaf-blind public transit riders. In *Proceedings of the SIGCHI conference on Human Factors in computing systems* (pp. 3247-3256). New York, NY: ACM Press. 10.1145/1978942.1979424

Bahadur, A. K., & Tripathi, N. (2016). Design of smart voice guiding and location indicator system for visually impaired and disabled person: The artificial vision system, GSM, GPRS, GPS, cloud computing. *International Journal of Current Trends in Engineering & Research*, 2, 29–35.

Behmer, J., & Knox, S. (2010). LocalEyes: Accessible GPS and points of interest. In *Proceedings of the 12th International ACM SIGACCESS Conference on Computers and Accessibility* (pp. 323-324). New York, NY: ACM. 10.1145/1878803.1878893

Bourne, R. R. A., Flaxman, S. R., Braithwaite, T., Cicinelli, M. V., Das, A., Jonas, J. B., ... Zheng, Y. (2017). Magnitude, temporal trends, and projections of the global prevalence of blindness and distance and near vision impairment: A systematic review and meta-analysis. *The Lancet. Global Health*, 5(9), e888–e897. doi:10.1016/S2214-109X(17)30293-0 PMID:28779882

Bradley, N., & Dunlop, M. (2008). *Navigation AT: Context-aware* computing. In M. A. Hersh & M. A. Johnson (Eds.), *Assistive technology for visually impaired and blind people* (pp. 231–260). Berlin: Springer. doi:10.1007/978-1-84628-867-8_7

Brito, D., Viana, T., Sousa, D., Lourenço, A., & Paiva, S. (2018). A mobile solution to help visually impaired people in public transports and in pedestrian walks. *International Journal of Sustainable Development and Planning*, 13(2), 281–293. doi:10.2495/SDP-V13-N2-281-293

Bujacz, M., & Baranski, P., & … Materka, A. (2008). Remote mobility and navigation aid for the visually disabled. In P. M. Sharkey, P. Lopes-dos-Santos, P. L. Weiss & A. L. Brooks (Eds.), *Proceedings of the 7th International Conference on Disability, Virtual Reality and Association Technologies with Art Abilitation* (pp. 263-270). Maia, Portugal: Academic Press.

Capella-McDonnall, M. E. (2007). The need for health promotion for adults who are visually impaired. *Journal of Visual Impairment & Blindness*, *20*(3), 133–145. doi:10.1177/0145482X0710100302

Carroll, T. (1961). *Blindness: what it is, what it does and how to live with it*. Boston, MA: Little, Brown and Company.

Cattaneo, Z., & Vecchi, T. (2011). *Blind vision: The neuroscience of visual impairment*. London: MIT Press. doi:10.7551/mitpress/9780262015035.001.0001

Chen, H. E., Lin, Y. Y., ... Wang, I. (2015). BlindNavi: A navigation app for the visually impaired smartphone user. In *Proceedings of the 33rd Annual ACM Conference Extended Abstracts on Human Factors in Computing Systems* (pp. 19-24). New York, NY: ACM. 10.1145/2702613.2726953

Cuturi, L. F., Aggius-Vella, E., Campus, C., Parmiggiani, A., & Gori, M. (2016). From science to technology: Orientation and mobility in blind children and adults. *Neuroscience and Biobehavioral Reviews*, *71*, 240–251. doi:10.1016/j.neubiorev.2016.08.019 PMID:27608959

Dobosz, K. (2016). Designing mobile applications for visually impaired people. In J. Estrada (Ed.), *Visually impaired: Assistive technologies, challenges and coping strategies*. New York, NY: Nova Science Publishers, Inc.

Dornhofer, M., Bischof, W., & Krajnc, E. (2014). *Comparison of Open Source routing services with OpenStreetMap Data for blind pedestrians*. Paper presented at the International Conference for Free and Open Source Software for Geospatial, Bremen, Germany.

Eimer, M. (2004). Multisensory integration: How visual experience shapes spatial perception. *Current Biology*, *14*(3), R115–R117. doi:10.1016/j.cub.2004.01.018 PMID:14986645

Engelbrektsson, P., Karlsson, M., Gallagher, B., Hunter, H., Petrie, H., & O'Neill, A. (2004). Developing a navigation aid for the frail and visually impaired. *Universal Access in the Information Society*, *3*(3), 194–201. doi:10.100710209-003-0088-0

Giudice, N. A., & Legge, G. E. (2008). Blind navigation and the role of technology. In A. Helal, M. Mokhtari, & B. Abdulrazak (Eds.), *Engineering handbook of smart technology for aging, disability, and independence* (pp. 479–500). Hoboken, NJ: John Wiley & Sons. doi:10.1002/9780470379424.ch25

Golledge, R. G., Klatzky, R. L., & Loomis, J. M. (1996). Cognitive mapping and wayfinding by adults without vision. In J. Portugali (Ed.), *The construction of cognitive maps* (pp. 215–246). Dordrecht, The Netherlands: Kluwer Academic Publishers. doi:10.1007/978-0-585-33485-1_10

Gori, M., Cappagli, G., Baud Bovy, G., & Finocchietti, S. (2017). Shape perception and navigation in blind adults. *Frontiers in Psychology*, *8*, 10. PMID:28144226

Gori, M., Cappagli, G., Tonelli, A., Baud-Bovy, G., & Finocchietti, S. (2016). Devices for visually impaired people: High technological devices with low user acceptance and no adaptability for children. *Neuroscience and Biobehavioral Reviews*, *69*, 79–88. doi:10.1016/j.neubiorev.2016.06.043 PMID:27484870

Griffin-Shirley, N., Banda, D. R., Ajuwon, P. M., Cheon, J., Lee, J., Park, H. R., & Lyngdoh, S. N. (2017). A survey on the use of mobile applications for people who are visually impaired. *Journal of Visual Impairment & Blindness*, *111*(4), 307–323. doi:10.1177/0145482X1711100402

Hakobyan, L., Lumsden, J., O'Sullivan, D., & Bartlett, H. (2013). Mobile assistive technologies for the visually impaired. *Survey of Ophthalmology*, *58*(6), 513–528. doi:10.1016/j.survophthal.2012.10.004 PMID:24054999

Harper, S., & Green, P. (2000). A travel flow and mobility framework for visually impaired travelers. In *Proceedings of the International Conference on Computers Helping People with Special Needs* (pp. 289-296). OCG Press.

Harrar, V., Aubin, S., Chebat, D.-R., ... Ptito, M. (2018). The multisensory blind brain. In E. Pissaloux & R. Velazquez (Eds.), *Mobility of visually impaired people: Fundamentals and ICT assistive technologies* (pp. 111–136). Cham: Springer International Publishing. doi:10.1007/978-3-319-54446-5_4

Hebler, S., Tuunanen, T., & Peffers, K. (2007). Blind user requirements engineering for mobile services. In *Proceedings of the 15th IEEE International Requirements Engineering Conference* (pp. 205-208). IEEE. 10.1109/RE.2007.56

Hersh, M. (2018a). Mobility technologies for blind, partially sighted and deafblind people: Design issues. In E. Pissaloux & R. Velazquez (Eds.), *Mobility of visually impaired people: Fundamentals and ICT assistive technologies* (pp. 377–409). Cham: Springer International Publishing. doi:10.1007/978-3-319-54446-5_13

Hersh, M. (2018b). Mobility, inclusion and exclusion. In E. Pissaloux & R. Velazquez (Eds.), *Mobility of visually impaired people: Fundamentals and ICT assistive technologies* (pp. 631–648). Cham: Springer International Publishing. doi:10.1007/978-3-319-54446-5_21

Hersh, M., & Johnson, M. A. (2008). Mobility: An overview. In M. Hersh & M. Johnson (Eds.), *Assistive technology for visually impaired and blind people* (pp. 167–208). London: Springer International Publishing. doi:10.1007/978-1-84628-867-8_5

Hill, E., & Ponder, P. (1976). *Orientation and mobility techniques: A guide for the practitioner*. New York, NY: American Foundation for the Blind.

Hoang, V. N., Nguyen, T.-H., Le, T.-L., Tran, T.-H., Vuong, T.-P., & Vuillerme, N. (2017). Obstacle detection and warning system for visually impaired people based on electrode matrix and mobile Kinect. *Vietnam Journal of Computer Science*, *4*(2), 71–83. doi:10.100740595-016-0075-z

ICT. (2018). *ICT 11: International Statistical Classification of Diseases*. World Health Organization.

Kaiser, J., Cmar, J., Rosen, S., & Anderson, D. (2018). *Scope of practice in orientation and mobility*. Association for Education and Rehabilitation of the Blind and Visually Impaired Orientation and Mobility Division IX.

Kane, S., Jayant, C., Wobbrock, J., & Ladner, R. (2009). Freedom to roam: A study of mobile device adoption and accessibility for people with visual and motor disabilities. In *Proceedings of the 11th International ACM SIGACCESS Conference on Computers and Accessibility* (pp. 115-122). New York, NY: ACM Press. 10.1145/1639642.1639663

Koutny, R., & Miesenberger, K. (2014). Virtual mobility trainer for visually impaired people. *Technology and Disability*, *26*, 211–219.

Lin, B.-S., Lee, C.-C., & Chiang, P.-Y. (2017). Simple smartphone-based guiding system for visually impaired people. *Sensors (Basel)*, *17*(6), E1371. doi:10.339017061371 PMID:28608811

Long, S. K., Karpinsky, N. D., Doner, H., & Still, J. D. (2016). Using a mobile application to help visually impaired individuals explore the outdoors. In G. Di Bucchianico & P. Kercher (Eds.), *Advances in Design for Inclusion* (pp. 213–226). Springer. doi:10.1007/978-3-319-41962-6_19

Loomis, J. M., Golledge, R. D., & Klatzky, R. L. (2001). GPS-based navigation systems for the visually impaired. In W. Barfield & T. Caudell (Eds.), *Fundamentals of wearable computers and augmented reality* (pp. 429–446). Mahwah, NJ: Lawrence Erlbaum Associates Publishers.

Loomis, J. M., Klatzky, R. L., Golledge, R. G., Cicinelli, J. G., Pellegrino, J. W., & Fry, P. A. (1993). Nonvisual navigation by blind and sighted: Assessment of path integration ability. *Journal of Experimental Psychology*, *122*(1), 73–91. doi:10.1037/0096-3445.122.1.73 PMID:8440978

Lopes, S., Vieira, J. M., Lopes, Ó. F. F., Rosa, P. R. M., & Dias, N. (2012). MobiFree: A set of electronic mobility aids fot the blind. *Procedia Computer Science*, *14*, 10–19. doi:10.1016/j.procs.2012.10.002

Lubin, A., & Deka, D. (2012). The role of public transportation as a job search mode: Lessons from a survey of persons with disabilities in New Jersey. *Transportation Research Record: Journal of the Transportation Research Board*, (2277): 90–97. doi:10.3141/2277-11

Martins, P., Mendes, D., & Paiva, S. (2016). Mobile platform for helping visually impaired citizens using public transportation: A case study in a Portuguese historic center. *International Journal of Emerging Research in Management & Technology*, *5*(6), 77–81.

Merabet, L. B., & Pascual-Leone, A. (2010). Neural reorganization following sensory loss: The opportunity of change. *Nature Reviews. Neuroscience*, *11*(1), 44–52. doi:10.1038/nrn2758 PMID:19935836

Minifie, D., & Coady, Y. (2009). Getting mobile with mobile devices: Using the web to improve transit accessibility. In *Proceedings of the International Cross-Disciplinary Conference on Web Accessibility* (pp. 123-132). New York: ACM Press. 10.1145/1535654.1535684

Moovit. (n.d.). Retrieved from https://www.company.moovit.com/about

Nakamura, T. (1997). Quantitative analysis of gait in the visually impaired. *Disability and Rehabilitation*, *19*(5), 194–197. doi:10.3109/09638289709166526 PMID:9184784

Novi, R. M. (1998). Orientation and mobility for sight deficient. In *Proceedings of the 9th International Mobility Conference: O&M moving into the twenty-first century* (pp. 88-91). Atlanta, GA: Rehabilitation Research and Development Center.

Overby, J. W., Woodruff, R. B., & Gardial, S. F. (2005). The influence of culture upon consumers' desired value perceptions: A research agenda. *Journal of Marketing*, *5*(2), 139–163.

Park, K., Goh, T., & So, H.-J. (2015). Toward accessible mobile application design: Developing mobile application accessibility guidelines for people with visual impairment. *Proceedings of HCI KOREA 2015* (pp. 31-38). Hanbit Media.

Purves, D., Augustine, G. J., FitzPatrick, D., & Williams, S. M. (2004). Neuroscience (3rd ed.). Sunderland, MA: Sinauer Associates.

Rieser, J. J., Guth, D. A., & Hill, E. W. (1986). Sensitivity to perspective structure while walking without vision. *Perception*, *15*(2), 173–188. doi:10.1068/p150173 PMID:3774488

Rimmer, J. H., & Braddock, D. (2002). Health promotion for people with physical, cognitive, and sensory disabilities: An emerging national priority. *American Journal of Health Promotion*, *16*(4), 220–224. doi:10.4278/0890-1171-16.4.220 PMID:11913327

Röder, B., & Rösler, F. (2003). The principle of brain plasticity. In R. H. Kluwe, G. Luer, & F. Rosler (Eds.), *Principles of learning and memory* (pp. 27–49). Basel: Birkhäuser/Springer Verlag. doi:10.1007/978-3-0348-8030-5_3

Rodriguez-Sanchez, M. C., & Martinez-Romo, J. (2017). GAWA – Manager for accessibility Wayfinding apps. *International Journal of Information Management*, *37*(6), 506–517. doi:10.1016/j.ijinfomgt.2017.05.011

Salive, M. E., Guralnik, J., Glynn, R. J., Christen, W., Wallace, R. B., & Ostfeld, A. M. (1994). Association of visual impairment with mobility and physical function. *Journal of the American Geriatrics Society*, *42*(3), 287–292. doi:10.1111/j.1532-5415.1994. tb01753.x PMID:8120313

Sánchez, J., Espinosa, M., & Merabet, L. B. (2013). Accessibility for people who are blind in public transportation systems. *Proceedings of the UbiComp*, *13*, 753–756.

Sánchez, J., & Oyarzún, C. (2008). Mobile audio assistance in bus transportation for the blind. *International Journal on Disability and Human Development: IJDHD*, *10*(4), 365–371.

Sánchez, J., & Sáenz, M. (2006). Assisting the mobilization through subway networks by users with visual disabilities. In P. Sharkey, T. Brooks, & S. Cobb (Eds.), *Proceedings of the Sixth International Conference on Disability, Virtual Reality and Associated Technologies* (pp. 183–190). Reading, UK: University of Reading.

Seemungal, B. M., Glasauer, S., Gresty, M. A., & Bronstein, A. (2007). Vestibular perception and navigation in the congenitally blind. *Journal of Neurophysiology*, 97(6), 4341–4356. doi:10.1152/jn.01321.2006 PMID:17392406

Sierra, J. S., & de Togores, J. S. R. (2012). Designing mobile apps for visually impaired and blind users - Using touch screen based mobile devices: iPhone/iPad. *Proceedings of the Fifth International Conference on Advances in Computer-Human Interactions*, 47-52.

Silva, C. (2017). *Criação de um manual de boas práticas para o desenvolvimento de aplicações móveis de apoio à mobilidade de pessoas com cegueira nos transportes públicos* (Unpublished master dissertation). Polytechnic Institute of Lisbon, Lisbon, Portugal.

Troancã, B., Butean, A., Moldoveanu, A., & Oana, B. (2015). Introducing basic geometric shapes to visually impaired people using a mobile app. In *Proceedings of the Romanian Conference on Human Computer Interaction* (pp. 91-94). MatrixRom Publishing House.

Tuttle, D. W., & Tuttle, N. R. (2004). *Self-esteem and adjusting with blindness: The process of responding to life's demands* (3rd ed.). Springfield, IL: Charles C Thomas.

Tuunanen, T. (2003). A new perspective on requirements elicitation methods. *Journal of Information Technology Theory and Application*, 5(3), 45–62.

ViaOpta Nav. (n.d.). Retrieved from https://www.viaopta-apps.com/Viaopta-navigator.html

WAI. (2018). *Mobile accessibility at W3C*. Available at: https://www.w3.org/WAI/standards-guidelines/mobile/

Wang, D., & Xiang, Z. (2012). The new landscape of travel: A comprehensive analysis of Smartphone apps. In M. Fuchs, F. Ricci, & L. Cantoni (Eds.), *Information and Communication Technologies in Tourism* (pp. 308–319). New York: Springer.

Wayfindr. (2018). *Open standard for audio-based wayfinding*. Retrieved from https://www.wayfindr.net/wp-content/uploads/2017/12/Wayfindr-Open-Standard-Rec-1.1.pdf

WHO. (2017). The future of eye care in a changing world. *Bulletin of the World Health Organization*, *95*. Retrieved from http://www.who.int/bulletin/volumes/95/10/17-202952/en/

WHO. (2018). *Blindness and vision impairment*. Retrieved from http://www.who.int/news-room/fact-sheets/detail/blindness-and-visual-impairment

Wong, S. (2018). Traveling with blindness: A qualitative space-time approach to understanding visual impairment and urban mobility. *Health & Place*, *49*, 85–92. doi:10.1016/j.healthplace.2017.11.009 PMID:29227886

Chapter 2
Strategies and Technology Aids for Teaching Science to Blind and Visually Impaired Students

Cristina Gehibie Reynaga-Peña
Tecnologico de Monterrey, Mexico

Carolina del Carmen López-Suero
iD https://orcid.org/0000-0003-0131-5760
Universidad Iberoamericana, Mexico

ABSTRACT

This chapter aims to provide a panorama of suitable teaching resources and strategies for science education of blind and visually impaired students. Although it is not a thorough review, its intention is to provide examples of what is possible to do specifically for experimental sciences (Biology, Chemistry, and Physics). The authors will also present the foundations for designing inclusive learning materials based on the user-centered design and universal design for learning (UDL) frameworks, using as example the development of technology-based tactile three-dimensional prototypes for teaching biology. An example of low-technology adaptations for making accessible instruments for the chemistry lab, using recycled materials will also be described, as well as adaptations for laboratory safety. Finally, there is also a section elaborating on the educational strategy to create inclusive and engaging environments in science laboratories.

DOI: 10.4018/978-1-5225-8539-8.ch002

INTRODUCTION

Inclusive education of students with visual disabilities, particularly with respect to science-learning activities, can be a challenge for teachers in the regular classroom. This is because traditional teaching mostly relies on visual resources that are not accessible to blind students, and are little illustrative for those with weak vision (López Suero et al., 2017). Currently, the prevailing resources for blind and visually impaired students available in schools are thermoformed vinyl graphics and Braille-printed texts, usually both have no color or text for sighted users. These resources are widely distributed because they are low cost; however, their use requires the learner to develop additional skills in order to interpret the information they try to convey, and certainly are not attractive for students who are sighted. This characteristic makes them non-suitable for their use in inclusive classroom environments. It then becomes important the development of novel resources specially designed for inclusive education, or the precise adaptation or improvement of existing materials, as an essential footstep to promote and facilitate inclusive science education.

This chapter aims to provide a panorama of suitable teaching resources and strategies for the inclusive science education of blind and visually impaired students. Mainly, it aims to provide examples of what is possible to do specifically regarding activities and experiments in the experimental sciences, such as those for Biology, Chemistry and Physics at the middle school or high school level. In terms of teaching resources and adaptations for inclusion, needed to carry on the curricula in regular classrooms, two design frameworks will be discussed. In particular, how they have been applied for the development of technology-based tactile three-dimensional prototypes for teaching biology. There are also suggestions on the educational strategy to be used by science teachers who aim to provide inclusive environments.

USER-CENTERED DESIGN AND UNIVERSAL DESIGN FOR LEARNING, TWO FRAMEWORKS TO FOSTER INCLUSIVE EDUCATION

User-centered design is a design philosophy and a variety of methods for creating products that meet the needs of the users; it takes into consideration their characteristics, needs, motivations and expectations. Indeed, the users should be involved in the design process either at specific times (prototype tests, interviews, feedback, observations) or as partners in the entire design process, in order for the design to be effective (Abras et al., 2004). In the case of a user-centered design focused in persons with disabilities, this implies knowing and understanding in depth their contexts, their activities, and the ways they communicate with their environment, in such way that the object produced is usable and satisfying for them (the users), in addition to being more effective for the purpose it is designed.

In terms of education, Universal Design for Learning (UDL) is the framework of choice to foster inclusive education, as it departs from the consideration that each individual, with or without disabilities, learns in different ways. UDL is grounded on three principles (Rose and Meyers, 2006): provide with multiple forms of representation, multiple forms of expression and multiple forms of engagement. Based on those principles, it has been proposed that implementation of UDL in classrooms benefits students with disabilities who major in STEM fields, as it provides them with alternatives in the materials, content and resources they use for learning (Izzo and Bauer, 2015). According to Rogers-Shaw et al. (2018), "Universal Design for Learning is a framework for the teaching-learning transaction that conceptualizes knowledge through learner-centered foci emphasizing accessibility, collaboration, and community".

In an ideal scenario to foster inclusive science education these frameworks can converge, with the main goal that all students participate with the same level of engagement and at the same time by having both, an accessible curriculum and accessible and inclusive learning resources to facilitate construction of knowledge. In other words, teaching resources should comply with the characteristics of being accessible for blind and visually impaired (designed for the blind as primary users), while they are also attractive and inclusive for individuals without such condition (designed under UDL principles). For example, educational materials using Braille could have color illustrations and regular printed text, or three-dimensional models should have the characteristics of tactile resolution favorable for blind people, but also hold contrasting colors while containing attractive visual information for persons with low vision or without visual impairment. In the same venue, materials that are more sophisticated could additionally provide auditory and visual information, plus other sensorial information such as smell, when appropriate. This way, the use of carefully designed educational resources under both of those frameworks, would not only allow full participation of visually impaired students in science lessons, but would also increase the opportunities for interaction with their sighted peers, because they would use the same learning materials.

SCIENCE EDUCATION FOR BLIND AND VISUALLY IMPAIRED (BVI) STUDENTS

In science, hands-on activities are essential for a meaningful learning. Since the 1970's, there have been reports on adaptations to make experiments accessible for the blind (Malone and De Luchhi, 1979), and several of them focused on chemistry experiments, mainly titrations (Hiemenz and Pfeiffer, 1972; Tallman, 1978). More recent examples of how researchers have shown that experiments on titration can be accessible by using olfactory cues, are the reports of Wood and Eddy (1996) or Neppel et al. (2005), demonstrating the use of the odor of raw onion, garlic or vanillin to indicate the endpoint of the titration of solutions of sodium hydroxide with hydrochloric acid. In those cases, odor is used instead of phenolphthalein, the most used color indicator of pH. More recently, Bandyopadhyay and Rathod (2017) have developed a more sophisticated adaptation, which is an android app to detect the color change of phenolphthalein at the titration end point. Other authors have also suggested the use of acoustics to evidence electrochemical reactions (Cady, 2014), or proposed the use of a program for sonification of space physics data (Candey et al., 2006).

However, there are also recent reports evidencing that it is usual that students who are blind are not allowed to perform experiments in the laboratory, but instead, are paired with a sighted student who performs the tasks and shares the information on the experiment that is taking place (Pence et al., 2003; Supalo et al., 2013). Opportunely, in the last few years, there have been organizations or groups that have offered science camps for blind and visually impaired youngsters (Wedler et al, 2014; Bech-Winchatz. & Riccobono, 2008) where hands-on experiences are enforced. We consider that, in order to seek a successful inclusion experience for BVI students, the incorporation of multi-sensorial activities and the use of teaching resources and materials carefully designed from the principles discussed in the above section is highly relevant. The same level of importance resides in the effective use of inclusive teaching strategies that promote active and autonomous learning by every student, which should happen in parallel to being able to offer laboratory activities with an experimental design that facilitates spatial cues for safe manipulation in the science laboratory. Below we describe some examples of educational materials and adaptations for the science classroom or laboratory, and the educational strategies we have used in experimental activities for blind students, as well as teacher development workshops.

Examples of Accessible and Inclusive Educational Materials and Instruments

Different groups have created and documented diverse tools to make the collection of scientific data accessible for BVI students; mainly, they have favored the use of available senses to convey information other than visually. Some authors have reported that tactile and haptic perceptions are a major way to communicate information for learning science and other subjects in formal and non-formal environments (Jones et al., 2006; Minogue and Jones, 2006). Such is the case of the tactile educational materials used to teach topics related to phenomena of light at the Museum of the Light in México City (Hernández and Contreras, 2007).

There are also devices designed to make accessible regular laboratory instruments via auditory information; meaning, these instruments can output their readings of data as sound rather than graphics or numbers in a digital display, as it usually happens. One of those instruments is the Talking LabQuest 2, a sensor interface for blind or low-vision students for use in science education, which uses Sci-Voice software. The Talking LabQuest 2 device couples to Vernier sensors (for pH, temperature, motion, conductivity, UV-Vis Spectrophotometer, etc), making their use accessible in such way that blind students can easily follow in real time chemistry and physics experiments (Supalo et al., 2014; Issacson et al., 2016). Using the Talking LabQuest 2, several experiments were adapted for the blind and the results were documented; some examples are the relation pressure-volume in a gas, an acid-base titration using a drop counter, and the study of exothermic and endothermic reactions (Kroes et al., 2016). Those studies report that some limitations were detected when several Talking LabQuest 2 were used at the same time, since it was hard for the BVI students to identify the voice of their own terminal. However, they also reported that after students got used to it, the technology helped teachers and students to create more inclusive environments, and promoted the interest in science fields (Kroes et al., 2016; Isaacson et al., 2016).

With respect to educational materials for the classroom, our group has developed tactile three-dimensional models to teach/learn biological concepts of microscopic nature (cell biology, microbiology, plant tissues), which are accessible to blind and visually impaired students (Reynaga-Peña, 2015). These models were conceptualized by scientists, so they have scientifically accurate information, and were developed by visual arts students, in order to be highly attractive to all learners. Because they were designed based on UDL principles, those 3D models hold adequate tactile resolution, contrasting colors and amicable tactile features (different textures, softness *vs* hardness, etc.) for blind students, while being engaging for sighted users as well.

The first generation of 3D models was further improved by adding touch-response technology to provide auditory information and hence promote autonomous learning. Prototypes were made using polymer clay, and then covered with silver paint that connected to sensors. The hardware to transduce the signal generated by touch was bought from Touch Graphics (www.touchgraphics.com). This way, the information reached a personal computer, triggering audio information through a special software developed specifically for each prototype. A highlight of this system is that each part of the 3D model was individually wired, so the scientific auditory information related to each part was displayed as the user touched it. In the 3D prototypes created this way, users can hear one, or many times, the audio descriptions containing scientific information regarding the topic that is being represented herein. This second generation of prototypes is innovative and even more engaging, but their production cost was high due to the technology used, the software produced for each of them, and their artisanal (hand-made) fabrication.

Commercial agencies, such as Touch Graphics, have also developed general touch-response materials and educational tools using technology, which can be used for science teaching/learning. Examples of those educational materials are 1) the Tactile Talking Tablet (TTT) device (Landau and Wells, 2003), where materials can be created for any subject and through the Authoring Tool software, those can be created by the BVI users themselves; and 2) the set of tactile graphics on STEM subjects, made on specially designed thermoformed vinyl, which hold auditory information. A highlight of the latter is a periodical table of the elements that contains colors and printed text, as well as Braille and tactile features. This table provides auditory information with the use of a smart pen, which reads codified patterns in the vinyl (http://touchgraphics.com/portfolio/ttpen-stem-binder/).

More recently, with the widespread use of 3D printing technology, there is a new trend to create and use 3D printed materials to substitute thermoformed graphics. Several examples in subjects such as Biology and Astronomy have been reported in the literature (Horowitz and Schultz, 2014; Grice et al., 2015). The possibility of using 3D printed objects versus 2D tactile thermoformed graphics is an advancement; however, most objects printed this way lack tactile resolution, particularly in terms of richness of textures, given that common 3D printers use a single type of printing materials. In addition, most -if not all- 3D printed materials, lack the technology that allow providing auditory information and therefore, do not promote autonomous learning. Thus, it is necessary to take into consideration the design frameworks we discussed in the above section in order to produce objects more suitable for users and for the educational goals they aim to reach.

Adaptations and Safety in the Experimental Sciences Laboratory

A crucial part in laboratory practices is seeking accessibility without losing safety. First, to help BVI students to work independently in the experimental sessions, a piece of tape can be placed in the shape of a cross to divide sections -as in a Cartesian plane- in the laboratory table, so students can identify where the materials and solutions are strategically located for experiments. The instructions for the experiment could be written in Braille for students to read, but also can be orally said at the time of the experiment. This strategy was used by our group in several workshops for blind participants (Reynaga-Peña et al., 2014) and in workshops for teachers (López Suero et al., 2017) in Mexico. In these workshops, each student was completely independent and was able to conduct the experiments in the regular time.

We also made low cost adaptations of devices for the chemistry laboratories using recycled materials. For example, to detect conduction current in chemical substances, an adapted device analogous to that commonly used in regular chemistry labs was built. In this device, which regularly uses a bulb that turns on when there is conductivity in substances, the bulb was replaced by a buzzer 3-4 kHz and 1.5-15 Vcc. The integrity of the user is protected by incorporating a recycled (old) cell phone charger to convert the output voltage of 110 V to 5 V. This way, the original device was easily converted to an accessible detection instrument, and thus, it became suitable for users with and without visual disabilities (López Suero et al., 2017).

When the laboratory is accessible and safe for all by using the measures described above, the teacher or lab instructor can direct students to do, in the same session, the regular experiments and the ones with adapted devices. This could also be an opportunity to share results, discuss ideas and more importantly, to create in this way an environment inclusive for all students.

The Educational Strategy Supporting the Resources and Materials

The key point in all learning experiences is the educational strategy for both, the classroom and the laboratory. Some of the first reports related to making science learning accessible to blind students were proposals highlighting the benefit of using multisensorial and hands-on activities (Malone and De Luchhi, 1979; Soler-Martí, 1999). Indeed, the benefits of multisensory learning are described with detail by Shams and Seitz (2008) who argue that "the human brain has evolved to learn and operate in natural environments in which behavior is often guided by information integrated across multiple sensory modalities" (p 412). This makes them conclude that multisensory protocols can better approximate natural settings and, as consequence, produce "greater and more efficient learning".

Our group has adopted the multi-sensorial strategy as well. Elsewhere, we have also described our experience of biology, chemistry and physics workshops for BVI students in Mexico, where we implemented multisensorial activities within a thoroughly designed instructional strategy to promote construction of knowledge by discovery and experimentation (Reynaga-Peña, 2014; Reynaga-Peña et al., 2014). The BVI students who participated in those non-formal science learning experiences reported they had fun and positive experiences; particularly, some expressed they have never performed experiments before, and stated "it was fantastic to be able to do things (by myself), because they (teachers) never let us touch anything" (Reynaga-Peña et al., 2014, p 16). A highlight of this report were also the statements of participants mentioning that they were able to work because the method was accessible to them, and even suggested that teachers working at all school levels should learn how to teach science to people with visual impairments.

In mainstream science classrooms, as well as in non-formal environments, an effective approach for teaching science is the Inquiry-Based Learning (reviewed by Minner et al., 2010). As a pedagogical strategy, inquiry-based learning fosters autonomy in students and helps develop generic skills by playing different roles during a science session. This constructivist strategy is based in questioning, observing, researching, analyzing and applying. All inquiry-based learning experiences have four essential stages: focalization, exploration, reflection and application; and students play specific roles to foster and assure collaborative work; these roles are secretary, reporter, leader and materials manager. At the beginning of the session, the teacher/facilitator will focus the group towards the learning objective in mind by making question(s) that the students will have to answer by exploration and experimentation. While the students explore and collect the evidence, they will have to organize to play the role assigned and to function as a team using their different abilities. In order for teachers to develop the skills necessary to promote inclusive science education using this strategy, we previously sensitize them with activities designed for this purpose (López Suero et al., 2017; Reynaga-Peña et al, 2018). In fact, awareness of the needs of students with visual impairments was a key element that induced a reflective dialogue between teachers about the importance of creating inclusive environments in science (Reynaga-Peña et al, 2018).

CONCLUSION

In summary, an ideal scenario to foster inclusion of students with visual impairments in mainstream science classrooms should be to hold lessons accessible and engaging for all students, including laboratory practices where BVI students can autonomously produce and collect data while using the same learning and experimentation materials as their sighted peers. This is possible through the production and use of teaching resources and curriculum which are suitable for all students. This is only possible when such resources are generated considering the frameworks of User-Centered Design and Universal Design for Learning.

REFERENCES

Abras, C., Maloney-Krichmar, D., & Preece, J. (2004). User-centered design. In W. Bainbridge (Ed.), *Encyclopedia of Human-Computer Interaction* (pp. 445–456). Thousand Oaks, CA: Sage Publications.

Bandyopadhyay, S., & Rathod, B. B. (2017). The Sound and Feel of titrations: A smartphone aid for color-blind and visually impaired students. *Journal of Chemical Education*, *94*(7), 946–949. doi:10.1021/acs.jchemed.7b00027

Bech-Winchatz, B., & Riccobono, M. (2008). Advancing Participation of Blind Students in Science, Technology, Engineering, and Math. *Advances in Space Research*, *42*(11), 1855–1858. doi:10.1016/j.asr.2007.05.080

Cady, S. G. (2014). Music Generated by a Zn/Cu Electrochemical Cell, a Lemon Cell, and a Solar Cell: A Demonstration for General Chemistry. *Journal of Chemical Education*, *91*(10), 1675–1678. doi:10.1021/ed400584m

Candey, R. M., Schertenleib, A. M., & Diaz Merced, W. L. (2006). Sonify sonification tool for space physics. In *Proceedings of the 12th International Conference for Auditory Displays* (pp. 289–290). London, UK: Academic Press.

Grice, N., Christian, C., Nota, A., & Greenfield, P. (2015). 3D Printing Technology: A Unique Way of Making Hubble Space Telescope Images Accessible to Non-Visual Learners. *J. of Blindness Innovation & Research*, *5*(1). doi:10.5241/5-66

Hernández, I., & Contreras, P. (2007). La luz a través de otros sentidos: Proyecto educativo surgido del entorno local [The light trough other senses: an educational project emerging from the local context]. In Memorias de la X Reunión de la Red de Popularización de la Ciencia y la Tecnología en América Latina y el Caribe (RED POP – UNESCO). San José, Costa Rica: Academic Press.

Hiemenz, P. C., & Pfeiffer, E. A. (1972). General Chemistry Experiment for the Blind. *Journal of Chemical Education*, *49*(4), 263–265. doi:10.1021/ed049p263 PMID:5016269

Horowitz, S. S., & Schultz, P. H. (2014). Printing Space: Using 3D Printing of Digital Terrain Models in Geosciences Education and Research. *Journal of Geoscience Education*, *62*(1), 138–145. doi:10.5408/13-031.1

Isaacson, M. D., Supalo, C. A., Michaels, M., & Roth, A. (2016). An Examination of Accessible Hands-on Science Learning Experiences, Self-confidence in One's Capacity to Function in the Sciences, and Motivation and Interest in Scientific Studies and Careers. *Journal of Science Education for Students with Disabilities*, *19*(1), 68–75.

Izzo, M. V., & Bauer, W. M. (2015). Universal design for learning: Enhancing achievement and employment of STEM students with disabilities. *Universal Access in the Information Society*, *14*(1), 17–27. doi:10.100710209-013-0332-1

Jones, M. G., Minogue, J., Oppewal, T., Cook, M., & Broadwel, B. (2006). Visualizing Without Vision at the Microscale: Students with Visual Impairments Explore Cells with Touch. *Journal of Science Education and Technology*, *15*(5), 345–351. doi:10.100710956-006-9022-6

Kroes, K. C., Lefler, D., Schmitt, A., & Supalo, C. A. (2016). Development of Accessible Laboratory Experiments for Students with Visual Impairments. *Journal of Science Education for Students with Disabilities*, *19*(1), 61–67.

Landau, S., & Wells, L. (2003). Merging tactile sensory input and audio data by means of the Talking Tactile Tablet. In *Proc. EuroHaptics '03* (pp. 414-418). IEEE.

López Suero, C., Reynaga-Peña, C. G., Lozano Garza, O. A., Sandoval Ríos, M., Dessens Félix, M., Ibargüengoitia, M., & Ibáñez-Cornejo, J. G. (2017). Ciencias experimentales en el aula inclusiva [Experimental sciences in the inclusive classroom]. In La práctica docente en la enseñanza de las ciencias. A práctica docente no ensino das ciencias [The teaching practice in the teaching of science] (pp. 59-65). Educación Editora.

Malone, L., & De Lucchi, L. (1979). Life Science for Visually Impaired Students. *Science and Children*, *16*(5), 29–31.

Minner, D. D., Jurist-Levy, A., & Century, J. (2010). Inquiry-Based Science Instruction-What is it and does it matter? Results from a Research Synthesis Years 1984 to 2002. *Journal of Research in Science Teaching*, *47*(4), 474–496. doi:10.1002/tea.20347

Minogue, J., & Jones, M. G. (2006). Haptics in Education: Exploring and untapped sensory modality. *Review of Educational Research*, *76*(3), 317–348. doi:10.3102/00346543076003317

Neppel, K., Oliver-Hoyo, M. T., Queen, C., & Reed, N. (2005). A Closer Look at Acid–Base Olfactory Titrations. *Journal of Chemical Education*, *82*(4), 607–610. doi:10.1021/ed082p607

Pence, L. E., Workman, H. J., & Riecke, P. (2003). Effective Laboratory Experiences for Students with Disabilities: The Role of a Student Laboratory Assistant. *Journal of Chemical Education*, *80*(3), 295–298. doi:10.1021/ed080p295

Reynaga-Peña, C. G. (2014). *Ciencia en el Aula Inclusiva. Propuesta didáctica: Los hongos, ejemplos de seres vivos* [Science in the inclusive classroom. Didactic proposal: Fungi as example of live beings]. Secretaría de Educación del Estado de Guanajuato, Centro de Investigación y de Estudios Avanzados del IPN.

Reynaga-Peña, C. G. (2015). A microscopic world at touch: Learning Biology with Novel 2.5 D and 3D Tactile Models. *Journal of Blindness Innovation and Research*, *5*(1). doi:10.5241/5-54

Reynaga-Peña, C. G., Hernández Valencia, I., Sánchez y Aguilera, E., López Suero, C. C., Ibargüengoitia, M., & Ibáñez Cornejo, J. G. (2014). Experiencias educativas en la enseñanza de las ciencias experimentales a niños y jóvenes con discapacidad visual [Educational experiences in the teaching of experimental sciences to children and Young people with visual disabilities]. In *Memorias del Congreso Iberoamericano de Ciencia, Tecnología, Innovación y Educación*. Buenos Aires, Argentina: Academic Press.

Reynaga-Peña, C. G., Sandoval-Ríos, M., Torres-Frías, J., López-Suero, C. C., Lozano Garza, O. A., Dessens Félix, M., ... Ibanez, J. (2018). Creating a dialogic environment for transformative science teaching practices: Towards an inclusive education for science. *Journal of Education for Teaching*, *44*(1), 44–57. doi:10.1080/02607476.2018.1422620

Rogers-Shaw, C., Carr-Chellman, D. J., & Choi, J. (2018). Universal Design for Learning: Guidelines for Accessible Online Instruction. *Adult Learning*, *29*(1), 20–31. doi:10.1177/1045159517735530

Rose, D. H., & Meyer, A. (2006). *A Practical Reader in Universal Design for Learning*. Cambridge, MA: Harvard Education Press.

Shams, L., & Seitz, A. R. (2008). Benefits of multisensory learning. *Trends in Cognitive Sciences*, *12*(11), 411–417. doi:10.1016/j.tics.2008.07.006 PMID:18805039

Soler Martí, M. A. (1999). *Didáctica multisensorial de las ciencias: un nuevo método para alumnos ciegos, deficientes visuales, y también sin problemas de vision* [Multisensorial didactics of the sciences: a new method for stodents who are blind, visually impaired and also without visual problems]. Barcelona: Ed. Paidós.

Supalo, C. A. (2013). The Next Generation Laboratory Interface for Students with Blindness or Low Vision in the Science Laboratory. *Journal of Science Education for Students with Disabilities*, *16*(1), 34–39. doi:10.14448/jsesd.05.0004

Supalo, C. A., Isaacson, M. D., & Lombardi, M. V. (2014). Making hands-on science learning accessible for students who are blind or have low vision. *Journal of Chemical Education*, *91*(2), 195–199. doi:10.1021/ed3000765

Tallman, D. E. (1978). A pH Titration Apparatus for the Blind Student. *Journal of Chemical Education*, *55*(9), 605–606. doi:10.1021/ed055p605

Wedler, H. B., Boyes, L., Davis, R. L., Flynn, D., Franz, A., Hamann, C. S., ... Wang, S. C. (2014). Nobody Can See Atoms: Science Camps Highlighting Approaches for Making Chemistry Accessible to Blind and Visually Impaired Students. *Journal of Chemical Education*, *91*(2), 188–19. doi:10.1021/ed300600p

Wood, J. T., & Eddy, R. M. (1996). Olfactory Titration. *Journal of Chemical Education*, *73*(3), 257. doi:10.1021/ed073p257

Chapter 3
Factors Determining Learning Object Quality for People With Visual Impairment:
Integrating a Service Approach

César Eduardo Velázquez Amador
*Universidad Autónoma de
Aguascalientes, Mexico*

Juan Pedro Cardona Salas
*Universidad Autónoma de
Aguascalientes, Mexico*

Jaime Muñoz Arteaga
*Universidad Autónoma de
Aguascalientes, Mexico*

Francisco Javier Álvarez Rodríguez
ⅈ https://orcid.org/0000-0001-6608-046X
*Universidad Autónoma de
Aguascalientes, Mexico*

María Dolores Torres Soto
*Universidad Autónoma de
Aguascalientes, Mexico*

Aurora Torres Soto
*Universidad Autónoma de
Aguascalientes, Mexico*

ABSTRACT

Determining the learning object quality presents a special complication because we must consider the characteristics of a software application and an instructional element; the above is complicated by the inclusion of the disability issue because there are factors that must be considered in a special way. The chapter has the objective of presenting which are the main factors that must be considered when developing learning objects for people with visual impairment. The instruments for determining learning object quality usually only consider the area expert perspective, without considering the user opinion. For the above, it is proposed to integrate aspects of service theory in the quality determination in order to generate learning objects that also provide greater satisfaction of use to the student. The chapter also presents example questions that can be used to assess the proposed quality factors.

DOI: 10.4018/978-1-5225-8539-8.ch003

INTRODUCTION

In order to properly start this chapter its necessary to define some basic concepts such as: Learning Object, Services Theory, Service, Service Quality and topics such as the application of e-learning to disability.

The term Learning Object (LO) was popularized in 1994 by Wayne Hodgins when he named the CedMA working group as "Learning Architectures, APIs and Learning Objects". There is not a fully accepted definition of the Learning Object term, a definition is: "It's a digital or non-digital entity, which can be used, reused or referenced during the learning supported by technology" (Aguilar, Zechinelli & Muñoz, 2003). There are 3 basic characteristics of a learning object: Accessibility, Reusability/Adaptability and Interoperability (Aguilar et al., 2003).

In the proposal, the Services Theory has been integrated, this with the purpose of closely linking the student (user) in the LO quality determination.

Because an LO is a software product, it is necessary to identify what quality aspects any software product must meet (Velázquez, 2007). The software quality is the fulfillment of the functionality and performance requirements explicitly established, of the development standards explicitly documented and the implicit characteristics expected of all professionally developed software (Pressman, 2006).

For the quality determination of the software component in a learning object, the ISO 9126 standard can be used (Velázquez, 2007). The quality factors of the ISO 9126 standard provide an excellent checklist to evaluate the quality of a system. The ISO 9126 standard identifies six key attributes of quality: Functionality, Reliability, Ease of use, Efficiency, Ease of maintenance and Portability (Pressman, 2006).

In the LO quality determination, the existence of technical, pedagogical, content and aesthetic and ergonomic aspects is distinguished (Velázquez, Muñoz, & Garza, 2007).

In relation to the technological elements are those that allow an LO to provide the advantages that are attributed to products made under the paradigm of object-oriented development such as reuse and adaptability (Velázquez, Muñoz & Alvarez, 2005); It is also necessary to consider the properties of any quality software, such as error-free operation (Velázquez et al., 2007).

Within the pedagogical elements are all those that facilitate the teaching-learning process such as the examples used and the possibility of experimentation and evaluation; only to name some of them (Velázquez et al., 2005).

In the content elements there are those that give information about the complexity of the topic and the level of detail with which the content is addressed (Velázquez et al., 2005).

The aesthetic and ergonomic aspects of an LO refers to the information presentation (sources, colors, size, in a few words all the elements of format) and the layout of it (symmetric or asymmetrical arrangement, use of positive and negative spaces and so on) (Velázquez et al., 2007).

The Services Theory refers to everything that is permanent and normal in the service production (Spohrer, Maglio, Bayley & Gruhl, 2007). Services can be defined as the application of competencies for the benefit of another, meaning that a service is a type of action, performance, or promise that is exchanged for value between the provider and the client (Spohrer et al., 2007).

Related to the service quality, this can be defined as the difference between the client's expectations about the service and the client's perceived service. If the expectations are greater than the performance, then the perceived quality is less than satisfactory and therefore the client experiences dissatisfaction (Parasuraman, Zeithaml, & Berry, 1985).

In the e-learning context, the students can be considered as the final client, since the satisfaction with an educational product / service is one of the consequences of the exchange between e-learning systems and students (Chen & Lin, 2007).

The use of a service-based approach in the creation of a model that explains the LOs quality is expected to provide a greater user satisfaction, the above because the evaluation will treat them not simply as a product, but as a service. The model presented in this chapter is linked to the services theory, this allows us to consider the point of view of the student, as was expressed by Jim Spohrer of the IBM Research Center in Almaden. "It is desirable that students, who experience the service of first hand use qualitative measures to measure the quality of service" (Spohrer et al., 2007).

E-learning or computer-mediated network learning has the potential to offer a high level of personalization for people with disabilities. Accessible e-learning is an attractive application that provides a critical goal for a large number of emerging information technologies, such as semantic web, intelligent agents, and adaptive web services (Treviranus & Roberts, 2006).

The optimization of individual learning for each student in an e-learning environment depends on one or both of the following components: (a) components that are transformable and / or (b) a sufficiently broad level of alternative components combined with mechanisms to match with the right components for the student (Treviranus & Roberts, 2006). The transformable components would include the following:

- User interfaces that support more than just conventional input and display devices (Conventional devices include the keyboard, mouse, screen and speakers).

- Content that may be susceptible to redesign, this must be sufficiently structured to allow reorganization and must contain adequate informational labels (metadata) in a way that allows us the reuse and rethinking (change of the purpose).
- The activities and applications that can be presented and controlled in a large number of ways and can be completed with a variety of contents.
- Learning management systems or knowledge management systems that implement a wide variety of ontologies and rules (Treviranus & Roberts, 2006).

If e-learning is designed and implemented correctly, it can effectively eliminate many of the barriers that students with disabilities have faced in traditional learning environments (Treviranus & Roberts, 2006).

Achieving the accessibility of people with disabilities to electronic educational resources, including learning objects, has been one of the objectives followed by several initiatives and organizations at the international level.

The guidelines of the Web Accessibility Initiative (WAI) are the result of the commitment adopted by the World Wide Web Consortium (W3C) to promote the use of Information and Communication Technologies (ICTs) among people with disabilities. Collaborating with organizations around the world, they are making a great effort to promote accessibility, mainly on the Internet through five main areas of work, research and development, which are: technology, guidelines, tools, education and contact. (Guenaga, Burger & Oliver, 2004), (W3C, 2017). Its best results are the publication and wide use of its guidelines:

- Guidelines for Web Content Accessibility 1.0 (WCAG) Explains in detail how to make a website accessible to people with a variety of disabilities.
- Accessibility Guidelines for Authoring Tools 1.0 (ATAG) For software developers, it explains how to make a variety of authoring tools the support for the production of accessible Web content, and also how to make the software development itself accessible.
- Accessibility Guidelines for User Agents 1.0 (UAAG) For software developers, it explains how to make accessible browsers, multimedia players and assistive technology that serves as an interface with the previous ones.
- Accessibility Guidelines for XML (XMLAG) For XML-based applications developers, it explains how to ensure that XML-based applications support accessibility (Guenaga et al., 2004).

The IMS Global Learning Consortium (IMS, 2019) has published specific guidelines for accessible learning and content applications developing. They have provided specifications to organize student information (System and enterprise Profiles from IMS), content exchange and measurement with any LMS (Content Packaging and Question and Test Interoperability from IMS) and describe learning resources created and used in different LMS (Metadata of Learning Resources from IMS) (Guenaga et al., 2004).

PROBLEM

Learning Objects are elements that due to their nature present special difficulties at evaluation, since they have both the characteristics of a software application and an instructional element (Velázquez, Muñoz, Álvarez & Garza, 2006).

The quality determination task in LOs has been addressed in different ways, one of the most popular is the use of instruments such as LORI (Nesbit, Belfer & Leacock, 2003), which allows this assessment from the area expert perspective, the problem with this evaluation is the lack of feedback from the user.

Other evaluation proposals present a group of instruments and process, that is the case of Erla´s Morales work (Morales, García, Barrón, Berlanga & López, 2005), but because it does not consider the student's point of view, the possibility of obtaining information on the deficiencies or errors detected by the user is lost (Velázquez, Muñoz, Álvarez, Pinales & Garza, 2008). In order to solve the previous problem, it has been proposed to integrate the Services Theory in the LOs Quality Determination.

The problem of the learning objects quality determining is even more complicated when we refers to people with visual impairment, since factors such as usability must be adapted to their disability. Some other quality elements, such as the adequate use of images and colors, lose meaning when their use are referring to a student with visual impairment, so the instruments to determine the quality that could normally be applied should be adapted considering the specific student disability.

Once a model that explains the quality in LOs integrating a service approach is defined, it is possible to determine the main factors to take in count to achieve greater satisfaction with people with visual impairment.

PROPOSAL AND RESULTS

To define a Learning Objects Quality Determination Model Integrating a Service Approach, in first place was necessary to make an extensive search of similar researches in books, electronic libraries, conference proceedings, grade works and Internet references, in which the Services Theory would have been integrated in the e-learning quality determination, but giving priority to the Learning Objects works. The most relevant articles found are presented in Table 1.

In the studies presented in Table 1 are addressed the Service Quality in e-learning and electronic services (No specific researches was found in the learning objects area in which the theory of services would have been considered). Once the search for similar works was finished, they were analyzed, with the purpose of making the formal proposal of the Model.

In the search for similar research to define the model only those that presented a measurement instrument, a model or another indication of the variables used were considered in the process. The search criteria for the related investigations were the following:

In first place, publications were searched for the keywords of learning objects, quality and service theory. With these search criteria no research was found in which the integration of the service theory as such was indicated, so the search criteria were modified.

Table 1. Research base studies

Base studies
Byoung-Chan Lee, Jeong-Ok Yoon e In Lee, Learners' acceptance of e-learning in South Korea: Theories and results (Byoung-Chan, Jeong-Ok, & In, 2009).
Parasuraman, Valarie A. Zeithaml y Arvind Malhotra, E-S-QUAL A Multiple-Item Scale for Assessing Electronic Service Quality (Parasuraman, Zeithaml, & Malhotra, 2005).
Emmanouil Stiakakis y Christos K. Georgiadis, E-service quality: comparing the perceptions of providers and customers (Stiakakis & Georgiadis, 2009).
Roach, V. y Lemasters L., Satisfaction with online learning: A comparative descriptive study (Roach & Lemasters, 2006).
Robin Kay y Liesel Knaack, Investigating the Use of Learning Objects for Secondary School Mathematics (Kay & Knaack, 2008).
DeLone W. H. y McLean E. R. T., The DeLone and McLean model of information systems success: A ten-year update (DeLone & McLean, 2003).
Mercado del Collado Ricardo y López Granados Mónica, Investigación institucional en el Instituto Consorcio Clavijero (Mercado del Collado & López, 2011).

Source: (IGI, 2014)

The next criterion used was the online learning satisfaction, which returned 11 investigations as a result. It is important to note that not all research was about learning objects, but focused on student satisfaction, which is a basic theme in service theory.

The e-Commerce success metrics were explored, obtaining a total of 6 investigations. Electronic services quality was considered with a total of 3 investigations. The service quality on websites was explored, obtaining a total of 2 investigations. Although not all of these investigations focused on educational resources, their main value was that they presented a greater detail in the integration of services theory in web systems.

Finally, the search focused on the learning objects use, finding a total of 5 investigations and in the e-learning adoption in which only one work will present its measurement instrument. These last works allowed deepening even more in the knowledge of the evaluation of learning objects, but they did not manage the services theory.

After analyzing the 28 researches found, it was concluded that only 7 of them were the most relevant, since they synthesized the variables presented in the 28 studies. The papers considered as the most relevant are those presented in Table 1.

The Model was originated with the intersection of the areas shown in Figure 1. Each studied area (E-learning Adoption, Service Quality in Web sites, Electronic Service Quality, Online learning Satisfaction, Learning Objects Use, e-Commerce

Figure 1. Areas consulted in the research
Source: (IGI, 2014)

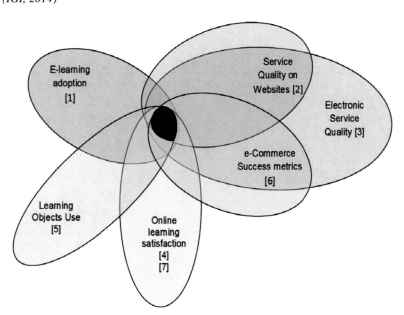

Success Metrics) has one or more investigations that have defined instruments for measuring satisfaction (Table 1), these studies serve as support for the model proposed in this research.

The Model is formed by the following independent constructors: System Quality, Information Quality, Service Quality and Playfullness and as part of the dependent elements we find the following constructors: LO Perceived Quality and Obtained Satisfaction (Figure 2).

The system quality constructor is formed by the following variables: Response time, Usability, Reliability, Availability and Security. The information quality constructor is formed by the following variables: Organization, Integrity, Ease of understanding, Relevance and Aesthetic Elements. The Service Quality constructor is formed by the following variables: help, interest and personalization (Figure 2).

The proposed model is designed to explain the quality of learning objects of aggregate type (large granularity), in which different learning, evaluation and collaboration activities are integrated.

In order to study the correlation on the constructors of the model, an instrument developed to determine the perceived importance on the proposed factors was applied. The application of the instrument was made at the end of 2011 to 41 students of the fifth semester of the Computer Systems Engineer career and 59 students in the first, fifth and seventh semesters of the Information Technology career from the

Figure 2. Model to Determine Learning Objects Quality Integrating a Service Approach
Source: (IGI, 2014)

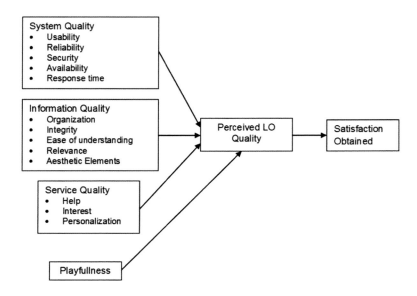

Autonomous University of Aguascalientes (UAA); Also 5 professors from different institutions (both national and foreign) with extensive experience in the development and use of LOs participated, to give a total of 105 participants.

For the application of the instrument it was necessary to be sure that the student had the knowledge of what is a Learning Object, for which a presentation on the subject was previously made, even if the student had previously worked with a LO.

To determine the perception of the importance of each factor, a 7 points Likert scale was used, 7 being completely important and 1 being completely unimportant. A 7 points scale was chosen because the application of the instrument was thought for university students and learning objects experts. The results were captured and analyzed with SPSS 12.

A correlation study was applied on the obtained data; from the data analysis a positive correlation was found among a large number of the variables. Then, a correlation study was applied on each of the constructors that define the Model, this with the purpose of determining the correlation coefficients and the critical level between the variables that make up each constructor.

It was found that all the questions from the Service Quality, Obtained Satisfaction, and Playfullness constructors present a significant linear relation to each other, that is, they are significantly correlated.

Most of the questions from the System Quality, Perceived Quality and Information Quality constructors present a significant linear relationship, so they are significantly correlated. The ranges of values in which the Pearson correlation coefficient are found per constructor are presented in Table 2.

Within the System Quality constructor, the Security variable was not correlated with the other variables and in the Information Quality constructor, the Aesthetic Elements variable was not correlated with seven constructor questions (out of a total of 14).

Table 2. Results of the Correlation Study on the constructors of the Initial Conceptual Model

Construtor	Value Range of the Pearson Correlation Coefficient
System Quality	0.27 a 0.44
Information Quality	0.19 a 0.47
LO Perceived Quality	0.34 a 0.62
Service Quality	0.25 a 0.57
Playfullness	0.28 a 0.44
Satisfaction Obtained	0.54

Source: (IGI, 2014)

A possible explanation for the lack of correlation of the Security variable may be due to the fact that Privacy (the protection of personal information) and Security (protection of users against the risks of fraud and financial losses) have been shown empirically to have a strong impact in the attitude towards the use of online financial services (Montoya-Weiss, Voss & Grewal, 2003), but this could be different for educational applications in which the user's priorities may vary.

Factors to Consider for People With Visual Disability

Consideration of all the factors of the proposed model increases the possibility of creating learning objects that provide greater satisfaction to the user, but to ensure the greatest degree of satisfaction with the learning objects by the users with visual impairment, it is necessary to provide greater attention to certain factors of System Quality and Service Quality. The Table 3 presents a description of the operational variables considered relevant for students with visual impairment.

Regarding the System Quality, the main factor to consider is the Usability. The elements of Usability must be adapted depending on the type of impairment presented, for example, in the case of blindness, it is possible to opt for the use of auditory resources or specialized hardware for presentation in Braille and for the

Table 3. Description of the operational variables considered relevant for students with visual impairment

Variable	Operational Definition
SYSTEM QUALITY	Degree of compliance with factors taken from the domain of software engineering, with which the operation is assured as easy, safe, adequate, fast and free of possible errors.
Usability	The degree to which students believe that the Learning Object will be easy to use.
SERVICE QUALITY	It is the degree of satisfaction that the student shows in relation to the service provided by the LO in aspects such as concern for their academic performance, help in the resolution of technical or pedagogical problems, the ability to adapt the resource to their needs and what So much work is enjoyed with the LO.
Support (Help)	It is the help provided to the student when encountering a technical or pedagogical problem. In some investigations it is equivalent to the concept of responsiveness, which is defined as the quick response and the possibility of obtaining help if there is a problem or question (Parasuraman et al., 2005).
Personalization	It is the ability to adapt the Electronic Educational Resource to the needs of the student. From an electronic commerce perspective, personalization is defined as how much and how easily the site can be adapted to the individual preferences of customers, stories and forms of purchase (Parasuraman et al., 2005).

Source: (IGI, 2014)

case of visual weakness, the handling of the usability may be different, since you have the possibility to increase the size of the text fonts.

Depending on the type of impairment, its degree and particular characteristics such as age or academic level, the resources that increase usability should change.

Related to Service Quality, the main factors to consider are Support (Help) and Personalization. Support refers to the help provided to the student when encountering a technical or pedagogical problem. It is proposed to measure this factor by the following questions: a) It offers help when a technical problem arises during the learning process. b) It offers help when a pedagogical problem arises during the learning process. c) The help functions are useful.

The Personalization is the ability to adapt the Learning Object to the needs or preferences of the student. It is proposed to measure this factor by the question: a) It allows to personalize my work with it. From an e-commerce perspective, personalization is defined as how much and how easily the site can be adapted to the individual preferences of customers, stories and forms of buy (Parasuraman et al., 2005).

Both elements, the Support and Personalization, must be adapted depending on the type of impairment presented. Table 4 presents the questions by constructor considered most relevant for students with visual impairment.

Table 4. List of questions by constructor considered most relevant for students with visual impairment

Constructor	Question
Usability	1.- It is easy to use and navigate in the LO.
	2.- It is easy to reach any part of the LO.
	3.- It is easy to find what I need in the LO.
Perceived Service Quality	1.- In general, I consider that the LO offers me the necessary services to learn
Support (Help)	1.- The LO offers me help when a technical problem arises during the learning process.
	2.- The LO offers me help when a pedagogical problem arises during the learning process.
	3.- The help functions in the LO were useful.
Personalization	1.- The LO allows me to personalize my work.

Source: (IGI, 2014)

CONCLUSION

In the chapter, a Model to Determine the Learning Objects Quality integrating a Service Approach (Figure 2) was presented, as well as the main studies that served as a basis to define it.

The importance of the proposal lies in the possibility of integrating the satisfaction of the user in the evaluation of LOs, achieving with this feedback the student to know some aspects that can escape the view of the evaluator, all with a view to improving these instructional resources.

Regarding the application of the model to people with visual impairment, the main factors that must be considered are Usability, Support (Help) and Personalization. The usability issue is one of the most explored in software engineering, but in relation to personalization there is still much to investigate for the benefit of people with disabilities.

Table 3 presents a description of the operational variables considered relevant for students with visual impairment, and Table 4 shows a list of questions by constructor considered the most relevant for students with visual impairment. From what was presented in the previous tables, the researcher on learning objects quality for people with visual impairment can have a solid base for the development of instruments that determine the LOs quality, considering a service approach.

FUTURE WORKS

As future work, it is planned to continue experimenting with the proposed instrument, in order to validate or improve it.

It is also contemplated to adapt the instrument for other types of educational resources and disabilities.

REFERENCES

Aguilar, J., Zechinelli, J., & Muñoz, J. (2003). Hacia la creación y administración de repositorios de objetos de aprendizaje. *IV Congreso Internacional de Ciencias de la Computación, ENC 2003*.

Byoung-Chan, L., Jeong-Ok, Y., & In, L. (2009). Learners' acceptance of e-learning in South Korea: Theories and results. *Computers & Education*, *53*(4), 1320–1329. doi:10.1016/j.compedu.2009.06.014

Chen, L. H., & Lin, C. (2007). Integrating Kano's model into E-learning satisfaction. Industrial Engineering and Engineering Management. *2007 IEEE International Conference*, 297-301.

DeLone, W. H., & McLean, E. R. T. (2003). The DeLone and McLean model of information systems success: A ten-year update. *Journal of Management Information Systems*, *19*(4), 9–30. doi:10.1080/07421222.2003.11045748

Guenaga, M. L., Burger, D., & Oliver, J. (2004). Accessibility for e-Learning Environments. In *International Conference on Computers for Handicapped Persons* (pp. 157-163). Springer.

IMS. (2019). *Guidelines for Developing Accessible Learning Applications*. Retrieved from http://www.imsglobal.org/accessibility

Kay, R., & Knaack, L. (2008). Investigating the Use of Learning Objects for Secondary School Mathematics. *Interdisciplinary Journal of E-Learning and Learning Objects*, *4*, 2008.

Mercado del Collado, R., & López Granados, M. (2011). *Investigación institucional en el Instituto Consorcio Clavijero*. 3er Congreso Virtual Educa México, "Evaluación, Equidad y Calidad en la Educación a Distancia", San Cristóbal de las Casas, Chiapas, México. Disponible en: http://www.libroselectronicos.unach.mx/virtual11/dr_mercado1/index.html

Montoya-Weiss, M. M., Voss, G. B., & Grewal, D. (2003). Determinants of Online Channel Use and Overall Satisfaction with a Relational, Multichannel Service Provider. *Journal of the Academy of Marketing Science*, *31*(4), 448–458. doi:10.1177/0092070303254408

Morales, E., García, F., Barrón, A., Berlanga, A., & López, C. (2005). *Propuesta de Evaluación de de Objetos de Aprendizaje, II Simposio Pluridisciplinar sobre Diseño, Evaluación y Descripción de Contenidos Educativos Reutilizables*. Barcelona: SPDECE.

Nesbit, J. C., Belfer, K., & Leacock, T. (2003). *Learning Object Review Instrument (LORI)*. User Manual. E-Learning Research and Assessment Network.

Parasuraman, A., Zeithaml, V. A., & Berry, L. L. (1985). A conceptual model of service quality and its implication. *Journal of Marketing*, *49*(Fall), 41–50. doi:10.1177/002224298504900403

Parasuraman, A., Zeithaml, V. A., & Malhotra, A. (2005). e-S-QUAL: A multiple-item scale for assessing electronic service quality. *Journal of Service Research*, *7*(3), 213–233. doi:10.1177/1094670504271156

Pressman, R. S. (2005). *Ingeniería de Software (5ᵗʰ ed.). Mc Graw Hill.*

Roach, V., & Lemasters, L. (2006). Satisfaction with online learning: A comparative descriptive study. *Journal of Interactive Online Learning*, *5*(3), 317–332.

Spohrer, J., Maglio, P. P., Bayley, J., & Gruhl, D. (2007). Steps Toward a Science of Service Systems. IEEE Computer Society. doi:10.1109/MC.2007.33

Stiakakis, E., & Georgiadis, C. K. (2009). E-service quality: Comparing the perceptions of providers and customers. *Managing Service Quality*, *19*(4), 410–430. doi:10.1108/09604520910971539

Treviranus, J., & Roberts, V. (2006). Inclusive E-learning. In *The international handbook of virtual learning environments* (pp. 469–495). Springer Netherlands. doi:10.1007/978-1-4020-3803-7_19

Velázquez, A. C. E., Muñoz, J., & Alvarez, F. (2005). La Importancia de la Definición de la Calidad del Contenido de un Objeto de Aprendizaje, Avances en la Ciencia de la Computación 2005. VI Encuentro Internacional de Ciencias de la Computación ENC 2005, Puebla, Puebla, México.

Velázquez, A. C. E., Muñoz, J., Álvarez, F., & Garza, L. (2006). La determinación de la Calidad del Contenido de un Objeto de Aprendizaje. VII Encuentro Internacional de Computación ENC'06, San Luis Potosí, México.

Velázquez, A. C. E., Muñoz, J., Álvarez, F., Pinales, F., & Garza, L. (2008). Estrategias de Gestión de la Calidad en el Desarrollo de Objetos de Aprendizaje. Tercera Conferencia Latinoamericana de Tecnologías de Objetos de Aprendizaje LACLO 2008, Aguascalientes, Aguascalientes, México.

Velázquez, A. C. E., Muñoz, J., & Garza, L. (2007). *Tecnología de Objetos de Aprendizaje, Capítulo VI La Calidad de los Objetos de Aprendizaje. In Primera Edición 2007. D.R. Universidad Autónoma de Aguascalientes y Universidad de Guadalajara. Editorial de la UAA* (pp. 129–170). Aguascalientes, Ags.

W3C. (2017). *Web Accessibility Initiative*. Retrieved from http://www.w3c.org/wai

Chapter 4
Logic Blocks:
Manual Assistive Technology for Visually Impaired Students

Giselle Lemos Lemos Schmidel Kautsky
ⓘD https://orcid.org/0000-0002-8867-4098
Universidade Federal do Espírito Santo, Brazil

Reginaldo Celio Sobrinho
Universidade Federal do Espírito Santo, Brazil

Edson Pantaleão
Universidade Federal do Espírito Santo, Brazil

ABSTRACT

This chapter presents perceptions resulting from a piece of a continuing education course developed in conjunction with basic education teachers whose goal was to adapt and analyze the use of the logic blocks as a manual assistive technology, aiming inclusive pedagogical practices in the work performed in regular classes intended for visually impaired people's enrollment. It is about a qualitative research, outlined as research formation. The data were obtained through reports and activities developed by teachers participating in a workshop stimulated during a training course. The analyses are supported by the presuppositions of figurational sociology of Norbert Elias. The results make it clear that the teachers consider organizing the assistive technology application as a tool for inclusive pedagogical practices.

DOI: 10.4018/978-1-5225-8539-8.ch004

INTRODUCTION

In this chapter, the results for a part of a research-training carried out in 2015 will be shared, focusing on the demystification of Assistive Technology for a group of teachers of the common class who worked with visually impaired students registered in Basic Education schools. The objective of this phase of the study was to provide teachers with a critical reflection on the need for didactic and pedagogical training to work professionally in the schools of the recent societies that count on the enrollment of students with disabilities.

The researchers reflections and discussions are organized in the dialogue with the literature that deals with the continuous formation for the use of new technologies in the Brazilian schools, the pedagogical possibilities of use and adaptation of the traditional materials for the educational practice, considering the diversity of social-educational context of the country and the social-historical process of the development of technology by the human species, as a necessary knowledge of life in society, as defended by Norbert Elias.

According to Elias (1998), humanity has always lived under the imminence of threats of a non-human nature and human disasters. However, in a long-standing historical-cultural process, men constituted a control over these threats through the development of knowledge, which afforded to them adequate means or technologies that minimized their limitations, enhanced their actions, and facilitated the development of their daily activities.

In this compilation, the convergence provided by the technological advancement or knowledge development during evolutionary process of the human race, promoted and still does, movements which modify the individual and social relational conducts in the civilization dynamics (Elias 2006). Cinema, for instance, is a result of a technological process that has changed the way people see and reproduce the world for over and above paintings or statics photographs, this way, possibly, giving rise to new prisms and a new sensitization on the experienced reality. As a dynamic space where individuals are constantly in interrelation (Elias, 1994a, 1998).

Thus, the researchers highlight that the period between 1983 and 1984 in Brazil indicates the official advent of computers in schools thanks to the creation of Ceie - Special Commission on Informatics for Education. At that time, there was a commitment to implement projects with the aim of making the use of this tool popular among teachers (Tajra, 2012). However, it was through training programs for teachers that informatics obtained a space in school education, through teacher training courses, after promulgation of Law 9.394 / 96 - Guidelines and Bases of National Education. This law defends technology as the domain of technological principles that govern modern production; encourages research and scientific research, determining the professional training associated with different forms of education, work, science and technology. (Brito & Purificação, 2011).

Yet, the authors understand cinematic art symbolic productions are a type of knowledge and synthesis which presents elements that can be set as a research source (apart from the peculiarities of knowledge in esthetic and scientific scope) since it favors the contact with knowledge from different fields (Almeida, 2011). These productions bring us closer to the knowledge about the creation and use of different technologies that have helped to control the calamities imminent to the human being.

Thus, in order to promote cinema as a knowledge source, it is quoted a part of the plot of 2001- A Space Odyssey (1968), from Stanley Kubrick, a sci-fi classic movie. In this film, we are taken to small tribes where the hominids lived and their everyday lives were spent trying to resist natural disasters and wild beasts. Then, without having a group purpose, one of them realizes that a bone can be a weapon as well as a tool to improve feeding-knowledge observed, learned, memorized and passed along for all in that group by the others of the species.

This situation shows that throughout the evolutionary trajectory human beings "have populated the planet by learning through experience and passing it along for generation to generation as knowledge", which is associated to Elias's constructions (1998, p. 299). In this manner, it can be stated that we have in fiction a contribution for us to comprehend the capacity of the human being to produce technologies as a set of knowledge pertinent to their natural reality, aiming to preserve their lives and, consequently, preserve our species.

This learning as a result of always renewed efforts made throughout human history has driven to men's humanization and engagement to their context. Therefore, we can note that technologies acquisition becomes necessary for individual's association to specific social groups. As an example, Elias (1994b) presents the idea of language acquisition, especially the oral communication in different human societies, as an experience resulting from the social interaction which delineates the individual's insertion into a singular group. According to Elias (1994b), the oral communication can be pointed out as a technology which has changed and intensified the relationship among humans and is understood as a result from an evolutionary rupture in the relationship between human being and the animals as well.

This way, in a nonlinear way, into the social-historical dynamics, man has constituted other sets of knowledge for the symbolic representation of oral communication like the typography and, in a temporal advancement, the invention of electronic means which has enabled new information and communication technologies, whose use keeping on contributing for values and new human behavior modification in different recent societies, among them, the school.

For sure, the outbreak of new information technologies, especially the computer as a teaching tool (Tajra, 2012), significantly influenced and still does, the educational practices. The authors classify computer as Assistive Technology since it enables to have an alternative to traditional methodologies for students having any kind of limitation, taking into consideration the multiplicity of activities that can be planned for educational practice in school through the use of new technologies as a pedagogical tool for teaching. It is supported on Brazilian conception implemented by *Comitê de Ajuda Técnica* (Technical Help Committee), 2009, which points out the assistive technologies as:

a knowledge area with interdisciplinary traits which comprises products, resources, methodologies, strategies, practices and services aiming to promote functionality related to the handicapped people's activity and participation as well as of those with restricted mobility, having as a goal their autonomy, independence, life quality and social inclusion. (Brazil, 2009, p.26)

Therefore, technology in Brazil is considered assistive when it is employed to help in the functional performance of some activities and can be represented by instruments or equipment like computer, for instance, which is the most common and the most employed assistive technological tool in schools (Bersch, 2017; Tajra, 2012). Although the assistive technology is a tool to help with the inclusion process of handicapped people in school and in society, has to be an awareness that it is just a tool that by no means replaces the teacher.

Yet, we evaluated the programs carried out by Education Ministry from the 90's were not able to afford the implementation of computer laboratories in all schools and either to guarantee the training for all active teachers and did not consider the matter of technical limitation of these professionals. Therefore, the lack of specific knowledge to use this tool was unfavorable to implement the use of the computer as assistive technology.

This situation makes us think about teachers' training and work conditions and gives rise to matters on teaching practice and on the technological and pedagogical challenges for committed employment of the tool along with the students who have in the assistive technology one more possibility to improve school knowledge. This did not mean teachers need to be experts in informatics but the practice in school demands the teachers to be aware, critical and selective users of the computer as a tool to achieve professional success concerning their choices enabling students to learn.

On that basis, it is made clear that the popularity of computer as a tool made it known almost like the only accessible technology in schools for the diverse assistive use provided in education process dynamics. However, due to the lack of didactic and technological knowledge for the development of pedagogical work by effective use of the machine, the authors warn about the need to extend the concept of assistive technology. Thus, in order to carry out a "research-training" along with a group of Basic Education teachers in Espirito Santo State- BRA, we rely on the *Comitê de Ajuda Técnica* (2007) concept, which points out assistive technologies as a diversity of practices that comprises "products, resources, methodologies, strategies, practices and services".

Following the purpose of this text, the aspects resulting from the research will be presented, which presupposes the continued formation of elementary school teachers from a public school in the city of Espírito Santo-BRA. The researchers affirm that the research in question was subsidized by Norbert Elias's theoretical-methodological contributions, mainly the concepts of interdependence, figuration and technicalization (Elias, 1994a, 2001, 2006).

The particularity of the elaborations proposed by Norbert Elias lies in the fact that he bases his discussion on the intertwining of political, social and economic issues and on the processes of individualization in a long historical perspective. In this sense, Elias is emphatic in saying that the concept of figuration includes "expressly human beings in their formation" (Elias, 2006, 25). And it is in this sense that, for him, the interdependencies of human beings constitute the core of social configurations. Thus, it is observed that the Eliasian sociological approach is engaged in the study of how the individuals that compose a certain figuration are constituted considering the relations that they establish among themselves.

In this way, figuration and interdependence are associated and linked concepts. Elias (2001, p. 150) points out that "the mode of mutual dependence varies according to the social needs that lead to new connections between people." In this sense, social representations should not be interpreted as independent connections of individuals. Complementarily, individuals cannot be looked at in isolation or closed in a space, but immersed in a network of dependence and interdependence (Elias, 2001).

For Elias (2006, p. 11), the process of technology "involves a humanity, the notion that people knew relatively little of the world without which they lived. According to Elias (2006), it is the process of knowledge that evolves as the man works for a better life, so that he is able to be sealed, in order to meet the needs of life. In order to do so, he clarifies that the human being improves his living conditions and satisfies his needs from the technique, thus confirming that the process of changing a society is evidenced much more in the way of developing his technique than the techniques concrete in themselves.

In theoretical-methodological terms, the research is of a qualitative nature, outlined as "research-training". The authors Longarezi and Silva (2013) characterize "research-training" as a perspective constituted by a dynamic that actively involves the researcher and the subjects of the research in the construction of answers to the questions lived in the contexts of the teaching performance. In this sense, research training "respects the diverse forms of knowledge that exist and, fundamentally, it is a process of political formation" (Longarezi & Silva, 2013, page 223). Following up the text, part of the experience of the "research-training" process developed with a group of Basic Education teachers will be described.

MANUAL ASSISTIVE TECHNOLOGY FOR VISUALLY IMPAIRED STUDENTS

This study is part of a Master's Degree investigation empiric basis, which discusses the construction of tactile models for teaching practice with visually impaired students (low sight or blind). The aim was to demystify the term "assistive technology" in an extension course by presenting it as a product or resource, planned according to the students' particularity without avoiding the proposed by the Decree No. 142, September 16th, 2006.

It is worth noting that we constituted the extension course stating its continuing training character by reflecting about possibilities for inclusive teaching outlining a political and ethical position that sustains the individual's potential to learn the social knowledge symbols of the historical moment as a presupposition for a decent personal and professional life.

Initially, the work was dissociated from the use of computer software, later, at the end of the course, it was shown to the teacher the possibility to associate the Math knowledge developed by the use of "Textured Logic Blocks" with an educational software named "Logic Blocks", made available by Education Ministry. However, in order to serve the visually impaired individual (low sight and blind), we warn it is necessary the use of screen reader, remembering that no matter how sophisticated the simulations produced in a computer screen are, these representations remain plain (Lorenzato, 2006), which does not dispense with the use of tactile materials for these students.

At first, it was rescued, in the course procedures, the history of a pedagogical tactile material set traditionally present at schools but forgotten by teachers in their everyday activities- golden material, abacus, tangram, and logic blocks. Perhaps, this negligence results from the computer technologies spread, considered a more facilitator path for the students to develop their learning when compared to traditional materials.

During the meetings, it was assumed that the use of tactile materials can make the math classes more dynamic and more comprehensible for the visually impaired student. Thus, by considering the material objective for conditions of teaching work in the reality of our schools, we understand the use of logic blocks as a possibility for manual assistive technology that allows the comprehension of some math concepts, besides providing inclusion movements in school, concerning the different games that can be created through the planning for the material use.

It is worth highlighting this material named logic blocks was developed in the 50's by the Hungarian mathematician Zoltan Paul Dienes, "aiming to teach the basic operations for Math learning, like the classification and correspondence" (Kautsky, 2016). It is a set of 48 pieces divided into three colors (yellow, blue and red), four shapes (circle, square, triangle and rectangle), two sizes (small and big) and two thicknesses (thick and slim). With this knowledge, the blocks were evaluated and deducted it is a pedagogical material which could be used by visually impaired students (low sight or blind) in order to learn concepts like shape, size, and thickness.

It cannot be missed the commitment with the inclusion in school, aiming to school for all who are enrolled in it. From this conception, teachers should point out possibilities to use the logic blocks, which the authors assume as a manual assistive technology. Considering what was observed before, researchers have organized an analysis of the use of logical blocks as a possibility for inclusive educational practice. The professional experience of the teachers made it possible to think about the use of these blocks in activities involving all the class and the discussions revealed that the blind student would find himself in disadvantage taking part in it since the teachers' instructions for this activity with the blocks generally occur from the traditional colors of the pieces: yellow, blue and red.

Therefore, by having a perspective of a work where all the students could be reunited, it was thought of an adaptation of this material into a tactile one which could really favor the math concept learning and also the real schooling and inclusion of the visually impaired students (low sight and blind). This adaptation demands the use of different texture involving the pieces. At the end of this adaptation, we had the following classification: blue/ smooth, yellow/ fuzzy and red/ rough.

In Figure 1, it is possible to visualize the manual assistive technology of "Textured Logic Blocks" – the adaptation of the traditional material, developed in the "research-training" process with the teachers who participated in the study. It is important to emphasize that each teacher has adopted a set of logical blocks, with the purpose of using it pedagogically in his classroom.

With the adapted material, it was suggested to the participating teachers plan activities involving math knowledge and the Textured Logic Blocks as manual assistive technology to meet their student's realities and presented them in the course in order to make all the participants trade ideas.

During the presentations, the teachers' considerations about the knowledge learned through the training meetings were evaluated, as well as the incidence of this knowledge in the context of the classroom. The evaluation of the learning process on assistive technology was positive, despite criticism about the short period of

Logic Blocks

Figure 1. Logic Blocks textured by the extension course teachers
Source: Kautsky, 2016.

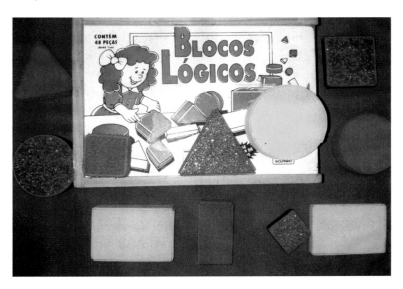

continuing training. However, in general, teachers reported that after the training meetings, it became a nuisance not to be able to fully develop their professional function - which is to teach, taking advantage of the materials available to the school. In this way, the analysis of the general evaluation of the training course shows that, in our social context, many teachers have the ethical commitment to provide access to school knowledge to all students who are under their responsibility (Kautsky, 2016).

CONCLUSION

The result of this work made the researchers reflect on the importance of the teacher's sight on their students as indispensable for construction and success of learning which includes: bringing credibility to their opinions, appreciating suggestions, observing, monitoring their development and understanding their singularities.

In this sense, it is understand that, although teachers should not restrict their practices to specific knowledge, the elucidation about the use of didactic resources, adapted to the singularities of the individual, as well as the use of methodologies and technologies that qualifies and potentiates the schooling of students with visual impairment is absolutely pertinent, since it can expand the possibilities of autonomy and inclusion of the person in social life outside of school.

Again, it is noted that the learning of a knowledge comprises an interaction between the people, just as it happened with the teachers during the dialogues in the continued formation undertaken. It is assumed that the use of intermediate instruments such as these textured blocks or other computerized assistive technologies that teachers have learned to master can contribute to the development of meaningful, pleasant and efficient learning, capable of arousing interest and motivation to seek knowledge and contribute to the learning. Learning the work of the teacher is the mediating basis of an important social right: scholar education.

REFERENCES

Almeida, R. R. (2011). *O Cinema como Itinerário de Formação*. São Paulo: Képos.

American Psychological Association. (2010). *Publication manual of the American Psychological Association*. Washington, DC: APA. Retirado de https://www.igi-global.com/publish/resources/image-guide.pdf

Bersch, R. (2017). *Introdução à tecnologia assistiva*. Porto Alegre: CEDI.

Brito, G.S., & Purificação, I. (2011). *Educação e novas tecnologias: um (re)pensar*. São Paulo: Ibpex.

Comitê de Ajudas Técnicas. Ata VII. (2009). Brasília: SDHPR - Secretaria Nacional de Promoção dos Direitos da Pessoa com Deficiência. Retirado de http://www.pessoacomdeficiencia.gov.br/app/publicacoes/tecnologia-assistiva

Elias, N. (1993). *O processo civilizador: formação do Estado e civilização*. Rio de Janeiro: Zahar.

Elias, N. (1994a). *A sociedade dos indivíduos*. Rio de Janeiro: Zahar.

Elias, N. (1994b). *Teoria simbólica*. Oeiras: Celta.

Elias, N. (1998). *Envolvimento e alienação*. Rio de Janeiro: Bertrand Brasil.

Elias, N. (2006). *Escritos & Ensaios: Estado, processo, opinião pública*. Rio de Janeiro: Zahar.

Kautsky, G. (2016). *A Formação Continuada de Professores do Ensino Comum no Campo da Educação Especial* (Dissertação de Mestrado). Universidade Federal do Espírito Santo. Retirado de http://repositorio.ufes.br/handle/10/8662?mode=full

Lei de Diretrizes e Bases da Educação Nacional de 1996. (1996). Brasília: MEC-Ministério da Educação e Cultura. Retirado de http://portal.mec.gov.br/seesp/arquivos/pdf/lei9394_ldbn1.pdf

Longarezi, A., & Silva, J. (2008). *Interface entre pesquisa e formação de professores: delimitando o conceito de pesquisa-formação.* São Paulo: Educere. Retirado de https://www.pucpr.br/eventos/educere/educere2008/anais/pdf/157_187.pdf

Lorenzato, S. (2006). *Laboratório de Ensino de Matemática na formação de professores.* São Paulo: Autores Associados.

Tajra, S. F. (2012). *Informática Na Educação: Novas Ferramentas Pedagógicas Para o Professor Na Atualidade.* São Paulo: Érica.

Chapter 5

Hedonic Utility Scale (HED/UT) Modified as a User Experience Evaluation Method of Performing Talkback Tutorial for Blind People

Eduardo Emmanuel Rodríguez López
Universidad Autónoma de Aguascalientes, Mexico

Jean Sandro Chery
Instituto Tecnológico de Morelia, Mexico

Teresita de Jesús Álvarez Robles
Universidad Veracruzana, Mexico

Francisco Javier Álvarez Rodríguez
 https://orcid.org/0000-0001-6608-046X
Universidad Autónoma de Aguascalientes, Mexico

ABSTRACT

Hedonic utility scale is a user experience (UX) evaluation method that, through a questionnaire, collects the hedonic and utilitarian dimensions of a product by rating items belonging to each dimension. In this chapter, it is proposed to adapt this method for its application with blind users using the Google TalkBack tutorial as a case study. Based on Nielsen's heuristics, five blind users rated the tutorial after completing each of its five tasks. To ensure inclusiveness in the adaptation of the method, this could be answered verbally and with the use of cards written in Braille, while, for questions of practicality in the evaluation, the number of items was reduced as well as changed the way of scoring (scale and equations) with respect to the original HED/UT. The scale of grades was ranked from 1 (very little) to 5 (quite), getting TalkBack scores between 4 and 5. The results show that the TalkBack tutorial is generally well accepted and well rated by users in both dimensions (hedonic and utility).

DOI: 10.4018/978-1-5225-8539-8.ch005

INTRODUCTION

In 2010, according to data from the World Health Organization, the estimated number of visually impaired people worldwide was close to 285 million, of whom 39 million were blind (OMS, 2017). In Latin America, 1 – 4% of population is blind (IAPB, 2014). Meanwhile in Mexico, according to figures from the same year, there were 1,292,201 people in the country with a limitation in activities to visualize, according to INEGI (INEGI).

The technological world is advancing by leaps and bounds, and human-computer interaction (HCI), *"a multidisciplinary research area focused on interaction modalities between humans and computers"* (Paolo Montuschi, 2014) is involved in everything humans do in everyday life. Although this progress is not entirely inclusive, since millions of applications are developed with any objective, from covering communication needs, to leisure or fun, without considering in equal measure, applications that can facilitate the lives of people with disabilities. This inequality can generate a digital divide, between people with access to all content (called info rich people) and people without access (called info poor people) (Villatoro & Silva, 2005). It is important to point out that as Cabero - Almenara says, *"the separation of communication technologies is becoming a reason for social exclusion and separation"* (Cabero-Almenara, 2008) therefore, actions must be taken to help minimize the digital divide (it should be clarified that there are several types of digital divide, such as access gap, gender gap, etc.).

There are important issues to mention that allow for a broader understanding of the relevance of the inclusion of people with disabilities in ICTs and fighting against digital divide:

- **Accessible technology**, that one *"that can be utilized effectively by people with disabilities, at the time they want to utilize the technology, without any modifications or accommodations"* (Lazar, Goldstein, & Taylor, 2015).
- **Digital empowerment**, *"empowerment of individuals and communities with information technology (that let people) gain new abilities and ways to participate and express themselves in a networked society"* (Mäkinen, 2006).
- **Digital competence**, *"DIGCOMP: A Framework for Developing and Understanding Digital Competence in Europe"* propose 5 competence areas which outline the key components of the digital competence, (see Table 1), (Ferrari, 2013).
- **Accessibility Acts**, for example the U.S. *"Twenty-First Century Communications and Video Accessibility Act (CVAA)"* that updates federal communications law to increase the access of persons with disabilities to modern communications (F.C.C, 2011).

Table 1. Digital competence areas

Competence Areas	Description
Information and data literacy	These ones deal with competences that can be retraced in terms of specific activities and uses.
Communication and collaboration	
Digital content creation	
Safety	There are "transversal" as they apply to any type of activity carried out through digital means.
Problem solving	

Source: Adapted from (Ferrari, 2013)

Although there are few applications developed for people with blindness disabilities, there are some important ones that can be emphasized, such as Talkback for Android or VoiceOver, a gesture-based screen reader that lets you use the Apple's device without seeing the screen (Apple, 2019), for iOS. The importance of these applications lies in their interaction with the blind user, through a narrator and the touch interaction that allows the user to open applications, activate elements, scroll through menus and even perform writing activities.

TalkBack is the Google screen reader included in Android devices. This function issues comments so you can use the device without looking at the screen (Google, 2018). The Talkback tutorial was the basis for evaluating the mobile application user experience using the Hedonic Utility Scale (HED/UT) method modified for blind individuals.

The method mentioned above, collects through a questionnaire, the pleasant and useful value of a service or a product. It uses a series of items of two different dimensions, the pleasant (or hedonic) dimension and the utilitarian dimension (Voss, Spangenberg, & Grohmann, 2003). The proposed modification of this method for use with blind people consists in granting a user-selected Braille or verbal weighting of each task in the Talkback tutorial on a scale of 1 to 5. This method was applied to five blind users based on the Nielsen heuristic.

METHOD SELECTION CRITERIA

AllaboutUX, an organization focused on UX measuring, propose a series of methods to evaluate all types of products and/or services (in this case mobile application) to know experience of users when interacting with them and then to can determine the quality of products, Check whether they really meet their objective or their feasibility, usability or functionality for users (Virpi et al., 2010). Therefore, using the following criteria: All methods that by themselves or by means of few adaptations can be applied easily to blind people do not necessarily require visual interaction or group work. We selected hedonic Utility Scale (HED/UT) method to be modified and to be used with blind users when evaluating the Talkback tutorial.

BACKGROUND: HEDONIC UTILITY SCALE (HED/UT)

In 1997, *"the first stage of a multi-phase process was presented to develop a generally applicable, reliable and valid scale for measuring the hedonic and utilitarian components (HED-UT) of attitudes"* (Spangenberg, Voss, & Crowley, 1997) In 2003 Voss, Spangenberg and Grohmann developed the hedonic/utilitarian scale method, which consists of the study of pleasant and useful value of a service or a product (Voss et al., 2003).

Procedures

- Ask the user, once a bran or a product has been selected, to choose one of the two characteristics of each item (from a list of 12 hedonic item and 12 utility items) according to their experience.
- Participation of the user is evaluated through statistical procedures.

In Table 2 the twelve utilitarian items and the twelve hedonic items with their positive and negative characteristics are presented.

The HED/UT has been applied in many different user experience studies, for example, *"Comparing text entry methods for interactive television applications"* a study *"to compare the user acceptance of alternative text input methods for an interactive TV application"* (Geleijnse, Aliakseyeu, & Sarroukh, 2009), or *"Beyond the wall of text: How information design can make contracts user-friendly"*, a study that *"investigates the unique contribution of layout and visual cues to the comprehension of complex texts"* (Passera, 2015).

As far as software is concerned, HED/UT was applied to evaluate the hedonic and utilitarian value of certain video games and their influence on product recommendation. The research results indicate that video games should be considered as both hedonic and utilitarian products and that the experience gained from playing them influences the hedonic and utilitarian dimensions and the desire to recommend the game to others (Storgårds, 2011).

This method was chosen because of its analytical aspect rather than evaluation, the convenience of evaluating two dimensions, hedonic and utilitarian. By evaluating both dimensions, we can get a global result of the user experience with this application.

Table 2. Hedonic & utility items

Utility items	Hedonic items
Effective / Ineffective	Fun / Not fun
Helpful / Unhelpful	Exciting/ Dull
Functional / Not functional	Delightful / Not delightful
Necessary / Unnecessary	Thrilling / Not thrilling
Practical / Impractical	Enjoyable / Unenjoyable
Beneficial / Harmful	Happy / Not happy
Useful / Useless	Pleasant / Unpleasant
Sensible / Not sensible	Playful / Not playful
Efficient / Inefficient	Cheerful / Not cheerful
Productive / Unproductive	Amusing / Not amusing
Handy / Not handy	Sensuous / Not sensuous
Problem solving / Not problem solving	Funny / Not funny

Source: Adapted from (Voss et al., 2003)

In addition, it can be done as a questionnaire. Significant modifications were done and will be presented in the next section.

DEVELOPMENT METHOD: HEDONIC UTILITY SCALE (HED/UT) MODIFIED FOR BLIND PEOPLE

Adjustments

The realized modifications to this method were made in terms of practicality to be used in blind people. Totally changed the way of qualifying the items, as well as their quantity, since some may be interpreted as repetitive or, may not be of interest sought in this study.

The first major difference with respect to the original method lies in the selected items and the use of only their positive characteristic, represented in Table 3.

The weighting that the user grants to each task is represented numerically with its equivalent description. The relationship between qualification and description is shown in Table 4.

As a first step, the hedonic and utilitarian grades of each task (CHT and CUT) are obtained. Subsequently, we obtain the average of each dimension (CFH and CFU) and the total product rating, which is the result of the average of the final hedonic and final utility grade (CGP).

Table 3. Selected items from the modified HED/UT method for blind users

Hedonic items	Utility items
Fun	Effective
Exciting	Helpful
Delightful	Functional
Thrilling	Necessary
Enjoyable	Practical
Happy	Beneficial
Pleasant	Useful
Cheerful	Handy
Amusing	Efficient

Source: Adapted from *(Voss et al., 2003)*

Table 4. Items classification scale

Score	Description
1	A Little bit
2	A little
3	Regular
4	A lot
5	Enough
Not Apply	Item does not apply

Source: Author's creation

Grades are obtained by the equations in Figure 1.
Where:

CHT: Hedonic task rating
CUT: Utility task rating
CFH: Final hedonic rating
CFU: Final utility rating
CGP: Overall product rating
calIH: Hedonic item rating
calIU: Utility item rating
n: Number of applied items
N: Number of tasks realized

Figure 1. Grade equations
Source: Author's creation

$$CHT = \frac{\sum_{i=1}^{n} callH(i)}{n}$$

$$CUT = \frac{\sum_{i=1}^{n} callU(i)}{n}$$

$$CFH = \frac{\sum_{i=1}^{n} CHT(i)}{n}$$

$$CFU = \frac{\sum_{i=1}^{n} CUT(i)}{N}$$

$$CGP = \frac{CFH + CFU}{2}$$

Note: "N" is considered as the number of tasks realized in the Talkback tutorial, because, depending on the Android device the blind people use, not always the five tasks of that tutorial can be realized.

As preferred by the user, two forms of evaluation of the modified HED/UT questionnaire are presented, either verbally or in Braille. Both forms of evaluation are expressed with the numerical qualification described below.

Verbal Method

After each task, the user proceeds to rate it. Numerically (1 - 5), the user verbally answers the qualification given to each item of both dimensions, which the evaluator questions him. Prior to the qualification, the evaluator explains to the user the relationship between qualification - description described in Table 3.

Braille Method

This method of evaluation is intended for users who know and are comfortable reading Braille. Likewise, at the end of each task, the user proceeds to rate it. By means of cards written in Braille (with a Perkins machine) and Spanish (for the evaluator to identify them), the user selects the one that he wishes to award as a qualification of each item for both dimensions (Table 3). Due to details of image quality of the cards (since they are made with self-adhesive mica for Braille writing), instead, a graphical representation of the "5" rating is shown in Figure 2. Enough ".

Figure 2. Graphical representation of the qualification 5. Enough
Source: Author's creation

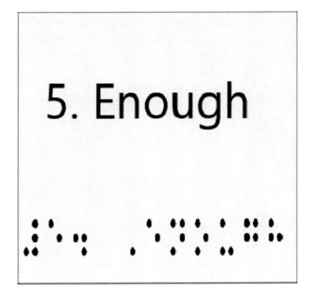

Definition of the Task and Evaluation Process

The task and evaluation process used in this research is summarized in five tasks to be carried out by the user. In the following, Table 5 shows in a simplified way, the tasks that the user performs in the Talkback tutorial.

Implementation

According to Nielsen's heuristics, in a study with Tom Lauder, *"The usability tests developed are a waste of resources. The best results come from testing no more than five users and running as many small tests as possible"*.

The Nielsen study found that when usability opinions are collected with a single test user, their opinions already cover nearly one-third of all usability errors that can be found. With the second user, there is some overlap, as he or she repeats some of the same things that the first user did, although new relevant information will be found, but not as much as with the first user. The third user will repeat many of the things that have already been found with the first and second user so only a small amount of new information will be added. As you go on testing with more users, you get less and less relevant information, so after five users, you will see the same findings again and again without learning anything new (Nielsen, 2000).

To perform this study, we have worked with five blind users willing to participate in the research to gather information about their experience in the Talkback tutorial. We worked together with the Institute "Desarrollo Integral de la Familia" (DIF) staff from the municipality of Aguascalientes for support in this activity. The flowchart shown in Figure 3, presents the procedure for applying the method.

Table 5. Talkback activities

Activity	Description
1	Basic navigation
2	Touch scroll
3	Talkback's Menus
4	Text Navigation
5	Edit text

Source: (Álvarez, Álvarez, & Benitez, 2019)

Figure 3. Flow diagram that represents the implementation of the HED/UT method with blind users for the Talkback tutorial
Source: Author's creation

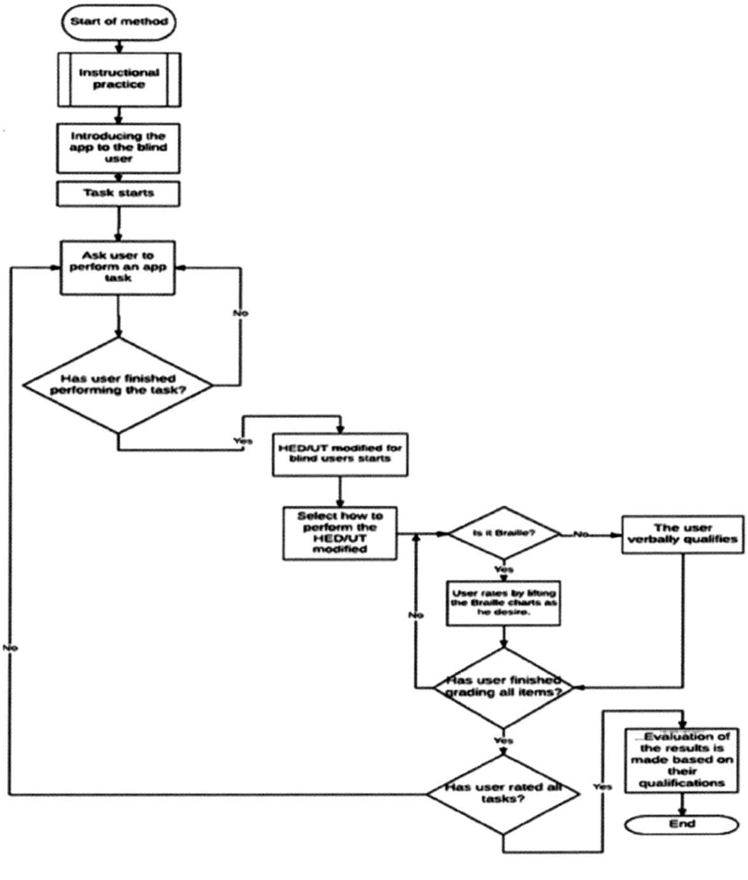

Final Evaluation Scale

The final product rating scale, that is to say, the scale interpreted by the CGP, is shown in Table 6.

Table 6. CGP's Interpretation scale

Score	Description
0 - 0.99	A little bit
1 - 1.99	a little
2 - 2.99	Regular
3 - 3.99	A lot
4 - 5	Enough

Source: Author's creation

RESULTS

Five blind users performed the Talkback tutorial and after each task the tutorial answered the modified HED/UT evaluation format. Four of the five participants chose to answer the assessment verbally, while the other in Braille.

For the sake of privacy, the identity of the users is not presented, they will only be referred to as User 1 to User 5. The results of their evaluation of each user's CFH, CFU and CGP are shown in Tables 7 to 11 respectively.

Table 7. User 1 evaluation rating

Ítems Hedónicos	Calificación					Ítems Utilitarios	Calificación				
	T1	T2	T3	T4	T5		T1	T2	T3	T4	T5
Divertido	5	5	3	NA	4	Efectivo	5	5	3	NA	5
Excitante	5	5	3	NA	4	De ayuda	5	5	5	NA	5
Atractivo	4	5	5	NA	5	Funcional	5	5	5	NA	5
Emocionante	4	5	1	NA	5	Necesario	5	5	5	NA	5
Disfrutable	5	5	3	NA	5	Práctico	5	5	1	NA	5
(Causa) Felicidad	5	5	1	NA	4	Benéfico	5	5	3	NA	5
(Causa) Placer	4	5	1	NA	4	Usable	5	5	5	NA	5
(Causa) Alegría	4	5	3	NA	4	Manejable	5	5	3	NA	5
Entretenido	3	5	3	NA	5	Eficiente	5	5	3	NA	5
CHT	4.33	5	2.6	NA	4.44	**CUT**	5	5	3.7	NA	5

Source: Author's creation

Table 8. User 1 Score: CFH, CFU & CGP

Score:	
CFH:	4.08
CFU:	4.67
CGP:	4.38

Source: Author's creation

Table 9. User 2: CFH, CFU & CGP

Score:	
CFH:	3.42
CFU:	4.17
CGP:	3.79

Source: Author's creation

Table 10. User 3 CFH, CFU & CGP

Score:	
CFH:	5
CFU:	5
CGP:	5

Source: Author's creation

Table 11. User 4: CFH, CFU & CGP

Score:	
CFH:	4.81
CFU:	4.92
CGP:	4.86

Source: Author's creation

User 1

As shown in Table 7, User 1 qualified each task and based on this, the CFH, CFU and CGP were obtained. The value obtained as a general product rating (CGP) by User 1 is 4.38, which can be considered as an "excellent" rating. According to the average he obtained in his hedonic ratings, his CFH was 4.08 and his CFU was 4.67.

User 2

Since the ratings of all tasks was performed in a similar way to User 1, only the results of the CFH, CFU and CGP are shown from this user. As shown in Table 9, User 2's scores were lower than User 1, in fact, his GPC was 3.79, which can be interpreted as "good". In turn, its CFH was 3.42 and its CFU was 4.17. It should be noted that this was the only user who decided to do the evaluation in Braille.

User 3

The ratings in Table 10 reflect that User 3 loved the Talkback tutorial so much that his CFH, FU and CGP was 5, which is understood as an "excellent" rating on the tutorial.

User 4

Table 11 shows the ratings of User 4, with a GFP of 4.86, a CFH of 4.81 and a CFU of 4.92, which explains the Talkback tutorial as "excellent".

User 5

As shown in Table 12, User 5 scored lower compared to others, with a CPG of 3.09, a CFH of 2.88 and a CFU of 3.29, even though, within the evaluation scale, the tutorial Talkback was rated "good".

DISCUSSIONS AND CONCLUSION

The results of the users were overwhelming, given that, according to their CGP, the Talkback tutorial rating is between "good" and "excellent". One aspect to emphasize is the evaluation of User 2, since it was the only one that chose the Braille

Table 12. User 5: CFH, CFU & CGP

Score:	
CFH:	2.88
CFU:	3.29
CGP:	3.09

Source: Author's creation

evaluation method for its domain of the same, and, therefore, the session lasted a little more than the average, that was between thirty and Forty minutes. It is also worth mentioning that User 2 rated the tutorial as "good" since, according to his words, "Talkback needs more tools". User 5 also rated the tutorial as "good," but the justification for his ratings is since he is not an Android user, he uses and has used the equivalent iOS software, VoiceOver, so he expressed his feeling in relation to which Talkback is not as complete as VoiceOver. In contrast to users 2 and 5, the rest rated the tutorial as excellent.

Another point to note is that, as shown in Table 8, Task 4 could not be performed due to problems in the mobile devices that were used to perform the tutorial. Similarly, this task could not be performed by other users for the same reasons.

As expected during the research, the modified HED/UT for blind people was able to quantify the Talkback tutorial. The ratings of hedonic and utilitarian dimensions show that Talkback has more affinity for a utilitarian sense than for pleasure or hedonic. This is because this tool is used to support applications that blind users cannot handle, so it is consistent that you have obtained a higher CFU.

This method of evaluation made it possible to observe and discuss how blind users interact with the tutorial, and what emotional relationship they find in it. For example, at the end of Task 5 (writing), they were questioned about how motivated they were to do it, and some users felt that the task was "excellent."

In relation to the utilitarian dimension, this method also allows knowing, for example, the practicality when performing a task on the part of the users. Recalling task 5 again, for some users, writing activities on the cell phone were not necessary or easy to do, which made them impractical.

After analyzing the user's qualifications when performing the Talkback tutorial, it can be asserted that using the Hedonic Utility Scale modified for blind people as a user experience evaluation tool, it is defined the functionality of the same.

The modified HED / UT represents an option to improve software developed for this type of users. Due to the nature of the method, it can be used to evaluate other software for the same cause.

FUTURE RESEARCH

- Exploración de métricas y modelos de aprendizaje orientadas a personas con discapacidad visual.
- Comparación de aprendizaje para personas con discapacidad visual y promedio mediante señales EEG.

REFERENCES

Álvarez, T., Álvarez, F., & Benitez, E. (2019). Proceso del método de evaluación de la usabilidad "pensando en voz alta" modificado y aplicado a usuarios ciegos en dispositivos móviles. *Dyna New Technologies, 6*, 12. doi:10.6036/NT9059

Apple. (2019). *Vision Accessibility - iPhone - Apple (CA)*. Retrieved from https://www.apple.com/ca/accessibility/iphone/vision/

Cabero-Almenara, J. (2008). *TICs para la igualdad: la brecha digital en la discapacidad.* Paper presented at the ANALES de la Universidad Metropolitana.

F.C.C. (2011). *21st Century Communications and Video Accessibility Act.* CVAA.

Ferrari, A. (2013). DIGCOMP: A framework for developing and understanding digital competence in Europe. Publications Office of the European Union Luxembourg.

Geleijnse, G., Aliakseyeu, D., & Sarroukh, E. (2009). Comparing text entry methods for interactive television applications. *Proceedings of the 7th European Conference on Interactive TV and Video.* 10.1145/1542084.1542112

Google. (2018). *Comienza a usar Android con TalkBack*. Retrieved from https://support.google.com/accessibility/android/answer/6283677?hl=es-419&ref_topic=3529932

IAPB. (2014). *Cifras de Ceguera en Latinoamérica*. Retrieved from https://vision2020la.wordpress.com/2014/07/14/cifras-de-ceguera-en-latinoamerica/

INEGI. (n.d.). *México en cifras*. Retrieved from http://www.beta.inegi.org.mx/app/areasgeograficas/default.aspx#tabMCcollapse-Indicadores

Lazar, J., Goldstein, D. F., & Taylor, A. (2015). *Ensuring digital accessibility through process and policy.* Morgan Kaufmann.

Mäkinen, M. (2006). Digital empowerment as a process for enhancing citizens' participation. *E-Learning and Digital Media*, *3*(3), 381–395. doi:10.2304/elea.2006.3.3.381

Montuschi, Lamberti, & Paravati. (2014). *Human-Computer Interaction: Present and Future Trends.* Retrieved from https://www.computer.org/web/computingnow/archive/september2014

Nielsen, J. (2000). *Why You Only Need to Test with 5 Users*. Retrieved from https://www.nngroup.com/articles/why-you-only-need-to-test-with-5-users/

OMS. (2017). *Ceguera y discapacidad visual*. Retrieved from http://www.who.int/es/news-room/fact-sheets/detail/blindness-and-visual-impairment

Passera, S. (2015). Beyond the Wall of Text: How Information Design Can Make Contracts User-Friendly. Cham: Academic Press.

Spangenberg, E. R., Voss, K. E., & Crowley, A. E. (1997). *Measuring the hedonic and utilitarian dimensions of attitude: A generally applicable scale*. ACR North American Advances.

Storgårds, J. H. (2011). *The Influence of the Hedonic and Utilitarian Value of Digital Games on Product Recommendation*. Paper presented at the AMCIS.

Villatoro, P., & Silva, A. (2005). *Estrategias, programas y experiencias de superación de la brecha digital y universalización del acceso a las nuevas tecnologías de información y comunicación (TIC): un panorama regional* (Vol. 101). United Nations Publications.

Virpi, R., Ming, L., Kari, P., Brenda, C., Arnold, V., Effie, L., ... Marianna, O. (2010). *All UX evaluation methods*. Retrieved from http://www.allaboutux.org/all-methods

Voss, K. E., Spangenberg, E. R., & Grohmann, B. (2003). Measuring the hedonic and utilitarian dimensions of consumer attitude. *JMR, Journal of Marketing Research*, *40*(3), 310–320. doi:10.1509/jmkr.40.3.310.19238

Section 2
Support Systems for the Blind and Visually Impaired

Chapter 6
Application Mobile Design for Blind People:
History Memorama

Alma L. Esparza Maldonado
https://orcid.org/0000-0003-4557-7455
Universidad Veracruzana, Mexico

Edgard Benítez-Guerrero
https://orcid.org/0000-0001-5844-4198
Universidad Veracruzana, Mexico

Alberto Montoya Bironche
Universidad Autónoma de Nayarit, Mexico

Carlos A. Medina Casillas
Universidad de Guadalajara, Mexico

Elizabeth Vazquez Garcia
https://orcid.org/0000-0002-4445-8764
Universidad Autónoma de Nayarit, Mexico

Jose F. De la Cruz
Universidad Autónoma de Nayarit, Mexico

Francisco Javier Álvarez Rodríguez
https://orcid.org/0000-0001-6608-046X
Universidad Autónoma de Aguascalientes, Mexico

Nephtali A. Hernandez
Universidad Autónoma de Nayarit, Mexico

ABSTRACT

The team software process is a methodology focused on software development on gears, which at the end of the construction ensures product quality. This quality must be taken into account for people with disabilities like visual impairment. According to World Health Organization, in a study conducted in 2010, the number of people with visual impairment in the world is around 285,389 million people, and in America, it is around 26,612 million. This chapter focuses on using the TSP for the construction of an application for people with visual disabilities, resulting in a quality product that will help in memory and, in addition, the user learns about the city of Aguascalientes, Mexico, allowing the inclusion of these users in society.

DOI: 10.4018/978-1-5225-8539-8.ch006

INTRODUCTION

Inclusion is a way to integrate a person into society so that he/she can participate, contribute and benefit during this process. The main objective of inclusion is that individuals, especially those who are in conditions of marginalization or segregation develop in the social field (Significados.com, 2017). As it is the case for people with disabilities.

The term disability, according to the International Classification of Functioning, Disability and Health, "are those who have one or more physical, mental, intellectual or sensory impairments and when interacting with different settings of the social environment may hinder their full and effective participation on equal terms to others" (Instituto Nacional de Estadística y Geografía, 2010). Conditions that should apply also in the use of technology.

Nowadays technologies, with the advantages they offer, good use should be given to them, but not necessary is given or taken advantage in the right way. The good use of technologies may help in various areas, for example, education, which allows teaching in an innovative way, to help improve the education of their students according to their specific needs. Therefore, it was chosen to design a game for people with visual disabilities that have completely lost their vision.

There are applications that are already designed for blind people, but most of them are readers of documents and even money, there are also games, but they have not been found many on mobile devices for the entertainment of people with visual disabilities and this teach history, develop memory skills and other, because for this disability is relevant the development of this skills (Sánchez, Flores, & Aravena, 2003).

The visual disability can be limited to people in performing everyday tasks and affecting their quality of life, as well as the potential for interaction with the world. Within the visual disability, according to the World Health Organization, there are different grades, such as blindness, moderate or severe vision loss, and low vision.

Blindness, the most severe form of visual disability, may reduce the ability of people to perform everyday tasks and walking without help. The rehabilitation of good quality allows people with various degrees of visual disabilities to enjoy life, achieve their goals and participate actively and productively in today's society.

There is a real need to have systems for people with visual disabilities to improve the mobility skills and orientation (TISE, 2009), it was therefore designed a game that even allows the user to have a form of distraction in order to speed up the ability to withhold information. This will allow the user to have a greater ease of memorization in their daily life, to put it into practice and have fun when doing it, allowing him to have a greater identification of his environment. In the updating of the ISO 9000:2000, the definition was as *"the degree to which a set of inherent characteristics meets the requirements"*

In order to achieve that the application meets these characteristics, it is necessary to develop an application with quality. The quality according to the ISO in the standard 8402:1994 defines it as the *"totality of properties and characteristics of a production process or service that gives its ability to satisfy stated and implied needs"*. In the updating of the ISO 9000:2000, the definition was as *"the degree to which a set of inherent characteristics meets the requirements"* (Echeverry, Cabrera, & Valencia Ayala, 2008). Especially in this last definition special emphasis is placed on meeting the requirements of consumers.

However, it can be contextualized on concentrating in different areas, for example for Deming, quality is more closely related to the internal processes of companies. *"The quality control does not mean perfection. It means getting an efficient production with the quality that is expected to obtain in the market."*. Nevertheless, For Joseph Juran the approach on quality management, in which he called it "Juran's trilogy" (Quality Planning, Quality Control and Quality Improvement) it expands the approach beyond the product and customer's satisfaction toward the quality in processes and the improvement of these in the general production: product, customer's satisfaction and processes involved (Penagos Granada, López Echeverry, & Villa Sánchez, 2016)

To ensure software quality, there are three important points to consider:

1. Software requirements which are the foundation of what measures the quality.
2. The specific standards which define a set of development criteria to guide the form in which software engineering is applied.
3. Implicit requirements that are not mentioned.

As it is mentioned above, the quality not only focuses on the product but also on the quality of the process that is used for the generation of this. Today, there are different development processes that focus on the generation of products that are agile methodologies such as Scrum, others that focus more on the documentation as RUP/UP in the designing part, and others such as the TSP that focus on the documentation and generate the product with quality.

The Team Software Process by its acronym TSP which is a process focused on software development throughout devices. This explains how and why it works, defines the teams and explain how it should work, it also attempts to solve the problems that may arise on the way to product development, as well as constant evaluation of the team (Humphrey, 2000). The TSP consists of 8 phases which are Beginning, Strategy, Planning, Requirements, Designing, Implementation, Testing and Postmortem.

This document explains the generation of an application, with the phases of the tsp, which fulfils the function of helping in strengthening the memory with a matchup that consists of placing cards on the table upside down and when one card is uncovered, the equal card must be matched. If it is not paired, it should be put in its place upside down, these cards are printed with representative locations of Aguascalientes, México, and tell its story, as it is the government building, Calvillo (a magical town), Rincon de Romos, cathedral, etc.; those services, in addition, to the teaching of the location of these places and its history.

METHODOLOGY

Applications that have been generated for people with visual disabilities are generally developed for the reading of the screen; however, their requirements are not only the reader, but it also requires entertainment applications, teachings, etc.

These types of applications usually present problems as (Fundación Auna, 2011)):

- Small Screen, insufficient contrast and not configurable for visually impaired.
- The menu contains an excessive number of functions and it is difficult to access.
- Deficiency in the ergonomics as reduced the size of terminals, small keys, heap and little perceptible to the touch.
- Translation from voice to data.

Besides, one of the features that people with visual disabilities require is shown in Table 1.

People with visual disabilities will need to strengthen the capacity to memorize because people tend to rely on a lot of things they learn, for example, learn the routes by which tend to walk by and have a security of not losing the route. They are also used to identify objects that are difficult to distinguish for example the container of yoghurt, in general, all have a similar shape, what varies is the labelling of the brand.

Blind people usually wear an order in things of daily life. This is due to the easy location that this generates, for example, "the third object to the left". Because of this, remembering is of utmost importance to be able to create a mental image of

Table 1. The main feature which must have an application for people with visual disabilities

Features	Definition
Management of synthesis of the own voice	The ability to provide the reading of texts that are displayed in the game would benefit blind people and individuals with low vision problems.

Source: (Fundación Auna, 2011)

82

the scene so these matchups are adequate to increase the learning of people and their ability to retention, from older adults to children, although it is also a hobby for all ages.

The development of applications that can use blind people helps them to not to feel ignored or rejected within the society they live in. Developing applications that help them find location, reading of texts, forms of communication with other people help to be included in addition to provide day-to-day activities. One of the main objectives for people who have a lack of vision is the access to culture and participation (García, 2009).

The authors Zappala, Köppel, and Suchocolski (Zappalá, Köppel, & Suchodolski, 2011) mention that the technologies in special education: "can facilitate a qualitative improvement in the teaching and learning processes, develop skills and competencies, respond to the uniqueness and to each student's individual needs and enhance motivations that will give a significant character to the learnings.

Special education is the modality of the educational system aimed at ensuring the right to education of people with temporary or permanent disabilities, at all levels. This refers to the development of projects in which new, innovative ways are integrated to improve and facilitate the learning of the same, an example is the use of technologies such as the use of audios, platforms, games, videos etc. for the improvement and development of skills.

That is why, taking into account the needs of people with visual disabilities, a game to be easy to use and understand was developed, but at the same time when the user plays he will develop little by little more than his capacity to withhold information, which is something that people in this condition need to develop enough to be able to have a greater agility of memorization and in this way feel included in the society that surrounds them, since it generates a sense of belonging with the people around them and avoids feeling excluded or isolated.

As it is complicated for people with disabilities to find the fact of being integrated, institutions have generated activities, projects and modalities that help people improve their quality of life and so that little by little it can be made that they feel integrated into society and with this their disability can be carried out in a more enjoyable manner in which the power of growing, developing and learning as a person will not be avoided.

The fact of providing a way to be able to interact better in their social environment for people with certain disabilities is that they should be aimed at the needs of each person according to his or her disability, taking into account what is what makes the person fails to be integrated in a comprehensive manner in their environment.

Besides the inclusion of people with disabilities in society, it is greatly important to take into account the inclusion, but in workplaces. People must also develop their skills and interact better, regarding the willing to implement their skills and generate a livelihood for their lives.

An example in Spain quoted by Fundación ONCE mentions that *"people with disabilities contribute to GDP almost in the same proportion than people without disabilities. In 2011, employed people with disabilities represented 1.84% of the total population and accounted for 1.83% of GDP."* (Fundación ONCE, 2015)

If people with disabilities are given opportunities for better integration as in their education to develop their skills, as in society for a personal and work setting, this will improve the status of people with conditions of disabilities.

As mentioned earlier, there are many games developed for people with different disabilities, but for a specific group of people such as those with visual disabilities there is not a lot of variety, and even more, when it comes to games on mobile devices. Most of the games are for computers and are based on auditory features, some examples of games are the following:

- **Blind Tales: Audio Adventures:** Blind Tales offered by TatosGames is a game where the audio has an important role to play. It was designed bearing in mind the possibility of playing with the vision. The controls are gestures and movements that have been designed to ensure the maximum involvement with the narrated world with the help of the compass and the one-touch screen. The game has been designed in order to be able to be played by people with visual disabilities, it is not Talk-Backed supported, so this function must be turned off before playing. The application is totally free and does not include advertising (TatosGames, 2014).

- **A Blind Legend:** It is the first game with a no-graphical interface for mobile devices in the category of action-adventure games, where the ears replaced the eyes. This game is fully accessible for people with disabilities, it is controlled by means of different screen gestures, primarily a virtual joystick.

Its history is based on the adventures of its character, Edward Blake, the famous blind knight. Guided by his daughter, Louis, which must find a way to get to the castle of the kingdom, avoiding any kind of pitfalls and confronting dangerous enemies. The application is free and without advertising (DOWINO, 2016).

- **Blindscape:** It is an experimental game of a narrated story which is completely developed through audio. The narrative is about the life of a man within an authoritarian society, which seeks to escape from its intolerable life, ending with it. The application does not include advertising and is completely free (Brown, 2016) (Brown, 2016).

- **Unobrain - Mental Games:** It is an application developed by the eleven (National Organization of the Spanish Blinds) and Vodafone foundation in Spain. Within its interface, the application allows access to different educational games. The free account allows users to play a session of 3 different games every 3 days. It does not include advertising. The Premium Account allows users to play a custom session of 3 games every day. Plus, all 60 available games are unlocked. The Unobrain application has adapted the TalkBack module, by which all sets come with narrative, being accessible for people with visual disabilities (Unobrain Neurotechnologies, 2016).

Based on the above, the problem is that doesn't exist application constructed for develop skills blind disability as the memory and consider the characteristics necessaries according to this disability like screen size, the menu, ergonomic, or to translate to voice, also, they work as a game and teach history and geography to Mexican people especially from Aguascalientes.

For application development was considered the phases of TSP which are explained in development chapter, and the elements necessary to construct the application, this phases consist in planning, requirement, design.

DEVELOPMENT

The game design was chosen to develop on the Android platform Studio for Android devices because the most people has a device that comes with the Android operating system.

For being a common operating system among people, this will generate a greater facility of use in the devices of the people, visually impaired users often use their devices with applications of reading and location, as it is the Talk-Back. This allows us to offer a form of distraction that they may also carry on their mobile devices.

Until the appearance of Android 4.0 (also known as Ice Cream Sandwich), the accessibility level of the operating system iOS exceeded Android. This has turned iPhone as the platform for smartphones of reference for blind users (Fernández & Álvarez, 2012).

Some of the features most visually impaired users use on mobile devices are shown in Table 2.

The use of TSP helps organizations establish a practice of mature and disciplined engineering to produce safe and reliable software in less time and lower costs (Chávez & González, 2011).

Table 2. Android's features

Feature	Definition
TalkBack	It is a simple screen reader, built on the speech synthesizer configured on the mobile device Android, which informs the user about location within the graphical interface and the events that occur in the interaction with the screen.
SoundBack	It is based on sounds that inform the event.
KickBack.	It is analogous to the above but based on optic stimuli.

Source: (Fernández & Álvarez, 2012)

According to Gomez, D. (Gómez, 2009), the TSP is a developmental process for teams of engineers based on CMMI, it helps shape equipment for the development of quality software.

TSP provides guidelines to help a team establish objectives, plan their processes and revise their work in order to enable the organization to establish advanced engineering practices and thus obtain efficient, reliable and quality products.

TSP is a solution based on processes to solve business problems, such as:

- Predictable cost and time
- Improvement of productivity and development cycles
- Improvement of quality products.

The TSP presents 5 roles which are:

- **Team leader:** Directs the team, ensures that all team members report their data in the processes and complete their work as planned. In addition, he conducts weekly reports on the progress of the team.
- **Planner:** Meets research planning, coordination and extension of activities according to the needs of the unit, by studying, developing and evaluating programs and projects in order to ensure consistency with the objectives of the institution.
- **Designer:** Is responsible for the creation of a system concept that will help meet the business objectives set by stakeholders, making sure that the site complies with the accessibility features, navigability, interactivity and usability to ensure a pleasant experience to the user (Villareal, 2016).
- **Developer:** a software developer is a programmer who focuses on carrying out elaborate stages of software development. The developer has a perspective or vision much more general on the project being carried out more in the application level that in the component level or in individual programming tasks (Geoservice, 2015). Something very important in software development

is the documentation of code. The developer is the one who knows more than anyone about the operation of the code, therefore, it is a great responsibility for him to document in a correct way the software code (Pérez, 2012).

- **Quality Staff:** Is responsible for ensuring the software product = Quality + time + within the cost (Jack Gido, 2012).
- **Support Staff:** The primary responsibility of this role is to make sure that the computer has the appropriate tools and needed methods for the project. It is expected that the support specialist collaborates with the development team of the project.

Once the roles and their objectives have been defined, it is presented below the construction of the product.

PLANNING

In the planning phase, the schedule of activities was elaborated, this is to keep track of tasks to be performed because there is a time limit (see Figure 1).

Requirements

The requirements were previously presented with the characteristics that must comply with the applications for people with visual impairments.

Figure 1. Schedule of activities
Source: (Authors)

Nombre de tarea	Duración	Comienzo	Fin
Definicion de proyecto	1 día	lun 19/06/17	lun 19/06/17
Planeación	4 días	mar 20/06/17	vie 23/06/17
Documentación	1 día	mar 20/06/17	mar 20/06/17
Requerimientos	1 día	mié 21/06/17	mié 21/06/17
Definición	1 día	jue 22/06/17	jue 22/06/17
Detalles y selección de herramientas	1 día	vie 23/06/17	vie 23/06/17
Diseño	5 días	lun 26/06/17	vie 30/06/17
Diagrama de Dominio	1 día	lun 26/06/17	lun 26/06/17
Diagrama de estados	3 días	mar 27/06/17	jue 29/06/17
Diagrama de actividades	3 días	mar 27/06/17	jue 29/06/17
Diagramas de casos de uso	3 días	mar 27/06/17	jue 29/06/17
Diseño de interfaces	1 día	vie 30/06/17	vie 30/06/17
Construccion	16 días	vie 30/06/17	vie 21/07/17
Interfaces	2 días	vie 30/06/17	lun 03/07/17
Elaboracion	15 días	lun 03/07/17	vie 21/07/17
Pruebas y correciones	6 días	lun 17/07/17	lun 24/07/17
Verificación	1 día	lun 17/07/17	lun 17/07/17
Correción	3 días	mar 18/07/17	jue 20/07/17
Pruebas de funcionamiento	2 días	vie 21/07/17	lun 24/07/17

Design

For the design phase, use case diagrams and entity relationship were carried out, in order to learn a little of how communication and interaction of the game with the user would be like, and the entities that the game would count with and its relationship with each one of the entities (See Figure 2 and Figure 3).

Once the diagrams are finished, the team started with the design of interfaces, the design of Fig. 4 was performed as a base, the first display indicates a space where the logo of the game will be placed followed by instructions that will be dictated to the user automatically once he enters the game. Then, the user will be indicated to use two buttons at the bottom of the cell phone, one on the left-hand side of a button to exit the game and one on the right side if the user has no doubt with the instructions he may enter the game by pressing the button.

The second screen shows how a list of options for the user to select a difficulty would be seen, in the home screen when the user selects "play" the interface will change where he will be dictated the existing difficulties and the order in which they are for the selection, and at the bottom there is a button to exit the interface and return to the homepage.

In the third screen, there is an exemplification of what the game would look like once the user selects the Play button on the Home screen and choose a difficulty of the selection, then he will be shown the arranged letters to start playing when the user wants to begin and at the bottom of the screen the Back button to return to the homepage screen.

Figure 2. Use case diagram
Source: (Authors)

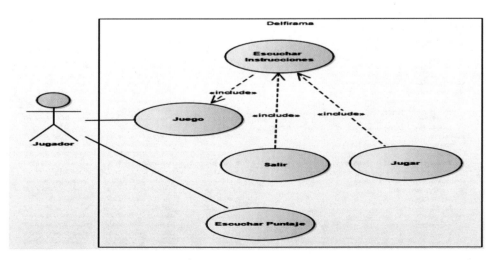

Figure 3. Entity relationship diagram
Source: (Authors)

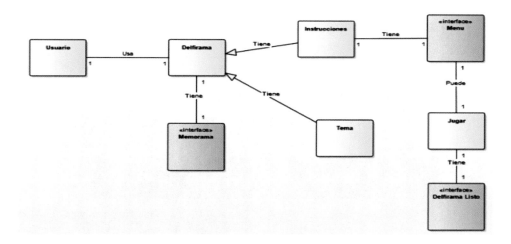

Figure 4. The interface design of the matchup application
Source: (Authors)

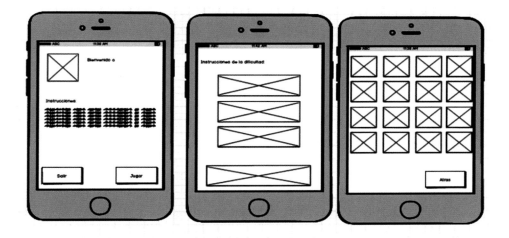

Implementation

Within the implementation of mobile devices cell phones were installed with Android v.4.2. The game (see Fig.5) consisted of buttons representing the card when pressing on it, it will emit a self-system sound, besides when entering the game, instructions are given in both written by those who are visually impaired, as in audio for those

Figure 5. Implementation of the application on the mobile device
Source: (Authors)

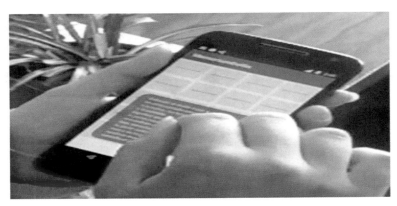

who are blind. When pressing the buttons and matching the pairs, a sound is played mentioning the story.

Each box of the game is mentioned by the number of the element and when flipping the card, the character belonging to it is mentioned, so that it can be identified and have space capabilities where each element can be (see Fig. 6).

Tests

To measure the quality of the generated application tests were carried out with blind users. The application is evaluated by means of questionnaires in which the important points are (see Fig.7):

- General Aspects (easy to use, motivating, instructions)
- Technical Analysis (use of different multimedia resources, quality of resources)
- Content Analysis (consistency between objectives and content, working area)
- Other aspects (motivates the user, beneficial learning)

The tests were conducted in the mobile application with eight blind users (see Fig. 8), according to Nielsen and Schneiderman, who say that apply test to five people can get results for usability measurement (Nielsen, 1955). And the tests were applied orally by the role of quality, this showed the results that were verbally exposed by the people.

Figure 6. Button functioning of the application
Source: (Authors)

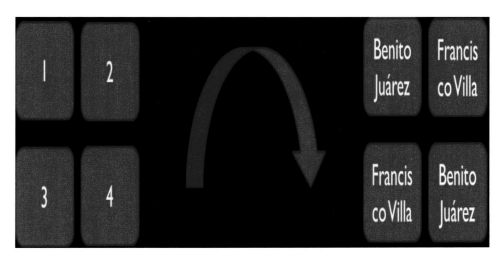

Figure 7. Evaluation of multimedia educational software
Source: (Gómez del Castillo Segurado M.T., 2017).

ASPECTOS GENERALES	M. M.	M.	R.	B.	M. B.	N. A.
Valoración general						
Elementos motivadores						
Aplicable a un amplio número de niveles						
Fácil de usar, no requiere adiestramiento específico						
El programa aporta instrucciones						
ANÁLISIS TÉCNICO						
Los gráficos son parte relevante del mensaje						
La imagen es parte relevante del mensaje						
La palabra en audio es parte relevante del mensaje						
El texto escrito es parte relevante del mensaje						
Utiliza percepciones multisensoriales						
Buena sincronización entre los elementos						
Calidad de los recursos multimedia						
ANÁLISIS DE CONTENIDOS						
Coherencia con los objetivos y contenidos						
Se especifican los objetivos de enseñanza						
Contenido actualizado						
OTROS ASPECTOS						
Favorece un aprendizaje activo y significativo						
Logra motivar al usuario						
Es beneficioso para el aprendizaje						
Cuenta con deversos niveles de dificultad						

RESULTS/QUALITY

According to the measurement in the system tests, the characteristics that the application should have to measure the quality of the application were assessed. As result of this measure, it was noted the fulfilment of the characteristics of Table 3.

Figure 8. Tests with users with blindness
Source: (Authors)

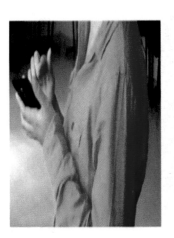 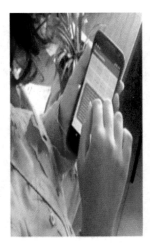 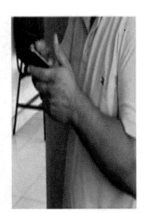

Table 3. The result of the compliance test of software features developed

GENERAL ASPECTS	V.G	G.	F.	B.	V.B	D.A
Overall rating		*				
Motivating elements		*				
Applicable to a wide range of levels		*				
Easy to use, does not require training	*					
The program gives instructions	*					
Technical Analysis						
Graphics are a relevant part of the message			*			
The image is relevant to the message			*			
The word in audio is a relevant part of the message	*					
The written word is a relevant part of the message		*				
Use multisensorial perceptions		*				
Good timing between the elements		*				
Quality of multimedia resources		*				

Source: (Authors)

Which mentions that it complied with most of the characteristics of the application, however, it showed errors and does not comply with the option of giving the score of hit rates.

With regard to the tests carried out with the user and the verbal test, results are shown in Table 4., which show that in general overall rating is well conceived, motivating elements are good, it is good to be applied to a wide number of levels, as a regular option it is that the graphics are a relevant part of the message, the image is relevant to the message, this as part of characteristics need to be covered by the software.

CONCLUSION

Performing this application presented several challenges as it was to meet t he features that people with disabilities require to carry out application development, the TSP follow-up as a process of development, as well as measuring the quality of the generated application. However, in spite of the challenges an application was developed to serve the role as entertainment, and at the same time that will support memory retention and teach the places and important people of the city of Aguascalientes. As a conclusion, when performing these types of applications, blind users will be benefited in their interactions and subsequently, this could serve as a role at work.

Table 4. Elements that were conceived into the software developed

	Action	Yes	No
Buttons	The buttons are of a considerable size which makes the users interact without difficulty	X	
Voice narrator	The voice of narration is clear and does not present any complications for the user's understanding	X	
Use instructions	Game instructions are clear and understandable.	X	
Game interaction	The interaction of the user and the program did not present any problem for the development of the same	X	
Errors	At the time of the execution of the program, failures and unforeseen events were found		X
Difficulties	The difficulties that were included in the game were in line with the section for location.	X	
Timing	It appears to be the option to add a late timing in order to undertake new challenges inside the game	X	
Score	It is indicated to add the option of a score of the game as a new challenge to overcome		X

Source: (Authors)

In addition, despite having carried out the TSP it became somewhat complex because it had too many different formats and documentation to generate in such a short time, without experience in this process, it was carried out what it was described in steps without generating the documentation required by this.

REFERENCES

Brown, G. (2016). *Blindscape*. Obtenido de https://play.google.com/store/apps/details?id=com.gavinbrown.blindscape&hl=es

Chávez, S., & González, C. (2011). *Team software process (tsp) sistemas de calidad en ti*. Obtenido de recuperado de: https://es.slideshare.net/silviachmn/tsp-

Dowino. (2016). *Blind legend*. Obtenido de https://play.google.com/store/apps/details?id=com.dowino.ablindlegend&hl=es

Echeverry, A., Cabrera, C., & Valencia Ayala, L. E. (2008). Introducción a la calidad de software. *Red de revistas científicas de américa latina y el caribe, españa y Portugal*. Retrieved from http://www.redalyc.org/articulo.oa?id=8920503058

Fernández, G., & Álvarez, F. (2012). *Juegos accesibles para juegos en plataformas móviles*. Obtenido de proyecto de sistemas informáticos.

Fundación Auna. (2011). *Las personas con discapacidad frente a las tecnologías de la información y las comunicaciones en españa*. Obtenido de fundación auna.

Fundación Once. (2015). Los beneficios de la inclusión social de las personas con discapacidad. *Cermi.es*. Obtenido de http://www.cermi.es/es-es/coleccionescermi/cermi.es/lists/coleccion/attachments/111/beneficios%20inclusion%20social.pdf

Geoservice. (2015). Obtenido de http://geoservice.igac.gov.co/mds/igac/ciaf/roles/desarrollador_igac.html

Gómez, D. (2009). *Team software process (tsp)*. Obtenido de http://alejandrogomeztsp.blogspot.mx/

Gómez del castillo segurado m.t. (2017). *Un ejemplo de evaluación de software educativo multimedia*. Universidad de Sevilla.

Humphrey, w. S. (2000). *Introduction to the team software process*. Addison-Wesley Professional.

Instituto Nacional de Estadística y Geografía. (2010). *Discapacidad en méxico.* (inegi) recuperado el 12 de oct de 2018, de http://cuentame.inegi.org.mx/poblacion/discapacidad.aspx?tema=p

Jack Gido, J. (2012). *Administración exitosa de proyectos.* Obtenido de cengage learning editores, s. A. De c.v.

Nielsen, J. (1955). 10 heuristics for user interface design. *World leaders in research-based user experience.*

Penagos Granada, E., López Echeverry, A., & Villa Sánchez, P. A. (2016). *Law on transparency implementation process.* ISO 27001 and Database Reporting on Public Entities.

Pérez, M. (2012). *Mario perez.* Obtenido de http://www.marioperez.com.mx/equipos-de-desarrollo/roles-y-responsabilidades/

Sánchez, J., Flores, H., & Aravena, G. (2003). Audiomemorice: desarrollo de la memoria de niños con discapacidad visual a través de audio. *Tise*, 1-25.

Significados.com. (2017). *Inclusión.* Recuperado el 10 de oct de 2018, de https://www.significados.com/inclusion/

Tatosgames. (2014). *Blid tales.* Obtenido de https://play.google.com/store/apps/details?id=com.tatos.blindtales&hl=es

Tise. (2009). *Actas xiv taller internacional de software educativo.* Tise.

Unobrain neurotechnologies. (2016). Obtenido de googleplay: https://play.google.com/store/apps/details?id=com.unobrain.gimnasio&hl=es

Villareal, C. (2016). *Perfiles y sus funciones en proyectos de tinorthware.* Obtenido de http://www.northware.mx/perfiles-y-sus-funciones-en-proyectos-de-ti/

Zappalá, D., Köppel, A., & Suchodolski, M. (2011). Incluso de tic en escuelas para alumnos con discapacidad visual. *Conectarigualdad.*

Chapter 7

Braille System Using an UX Evaluation Methodology Focused on the Use of Methods for Blind Users

Vanessa Villalpando Serna
Universidad Autónoma de Aguascalientes, Mexico

Jorge E. Herrera
Universidad Autónoma de Aguascalientes, Mexico

Teresita de Jesús Álvarez Robles
Universidad Veracruzana, Mexico

Francisco Javier Álvarez Rodríguez
ⓘD https://orcid.org/0000-0001-6608-046X
Universidad Autónoma de Aguascalientes, Mexico

ABSTRACT

Recently, technology has been advancing and making some aspects of life simpler. Most people have an intelligent mobile device. These devices have applications that support users to perform various tasks. However, these applications are developed for users who don't have any type of disability. This chapter focuses on making use of some tools that exist within the area of software engineering (SE) and user experience (UX) with the aim of developing an interactive software system (ISS). It is expected that this ISS will support people with visual disabilities to learn Braille. To develop the ISS, the authors use modified usability and UX evaluation methods for blind people. The methodology to be followed is based on the ISO15288: 2015 standard of the SE. The methods used to perform the evaluation tests with blind users are card sorting and thinking aloud. Based on the results, it is observed that the ISS complies with most of the UX factors, such as ease of use, accessibility, and utility, so they expect the ISS to be usable for blind people.

DOI: 10.4018/978-1-5225-8539-8.ch007

INTRODUCTION

According to Álvarez, T. (2018) there are currently few software development methodologies that involve a user with a disability and that at the same time focus on usability and UX. That is, there are few methodologies that focus on including users with visual impairment in the process of evaluating software engineering (SE).

The objective of this work is to develop an ISS focused on blind people and that this system complies with the UX factors.

To achieve compliance with the UX factors, we make use of an evaluation methodology of the UX for ISS with blind users proposed by Álvarez, T. (2018).

This methodology includes the stages of Analysis, Design, Development and Testing for the development and testing of the ISS. At each stage a modified evaluation method can be applied in order to make the ISS useful for the end user and be able to perform the test.

During the development process of the SE, two of the proposed modified methods were used: Thinking Aloud and Card Sorting. These methods allowed us to evaluate the UX factors and the ease of use of the ISS.

For the development of an ISS blind users must participate from the beginning of the tests to develop applications that are useful, usable and accessible to them.

It makes use of the methodology proposed by Álvarez, T. (2018), since it involves blind users from the initial stage of analysis to the delivery of the final product. Based on the above, the proposals and opinions of blind people are taken into account, crossing opinions with software developers, as indicated by the methodology.

It is important to involve the blind user from the beginning to make the relevant changes in the initial stages of development.

Based on the use of this methodology, it is expected that the final result of the ISS will meet the necessary characteristics to be usable and useful for blind users, that is, that the ISS for learning Braille will be simple and easy to use for blind users thus fulfilling with the basic factors of the UX.

STATE OF ART

Pérez & Gardey (2008) define the method as a means used to "reach something"; Aguilera Hintelholher (2013) defines the methodology as a term composed of the Greek words "methods" which means procedures and "logos" which means agreement.

Together these words result in the discipline that studies, analyzes, promotes and refines the method.

Regarding the term UX, Arhippainen and Tähti (2003) define it as the experience that the user obtains when interacting with a product under particular conditions, in another work Arhippainen (2003) defines it as the user's emotions and expectations and their relationship with other people and the context of use.

On the other hand, Nielsen and Loranger (2006) indicate that usability can be defined as ease of use. Specifically, it refers to the speed with which one can learn to use something, the efficiency when using it, what is its degree of propensity to error and how much the user likes it.

For these reasons, it is considered that UX and ease of use are one of the most important factors when evaluating the quality of an application.

The quality depends on the user have a positive and comforting perception when use the ISS taking into account that it is easy to use to ensure that the objective of the UX is met.

According to Álvarez, T. (2018), there are currently different methodologies focused on usability to develop ISS, however, most of these methodologies are focused on people with vision and are few that focus on users with visual impairment.

In general, the existing methodologies do not evaluate the UX, for example, Álvarez, T. (2018), mentions MPIu + a de Granollers et al. (2005), which is responsible for developing interactive systems that integrate aspects of usability in the SE life cycle related to accessibility for people with different disabilities; this methodology in Álvarez, T. (2018) is not considered viable because it does not determine the number of evaluations that must be carried out in a system, nor does it specify which methods should be performed or how many users or evaluators should participate.

It is also mentioned that following different types of methodologies have been developed desktop interfaces focused on people with visual impairment, as is the case of Sánchez (2010), Sánchez et al. (2009), Mioduser and Lahav (2004).

However, they mention that in spite of obtaining favorable results in each of the works, they do not focus on evaluating the usability of the product and independently of this point, it makes clear that they have been developed for desktop interfaces, therefore, what could have worked for a blind user in a desktop interface is not useful in a mobile interface.

For this reason, it was decided to work with the methodology proposed by Álvarez T. (2018) since we can evaluate usability and UX following the methods proposed in the SE for mobile ISS development, which focuses on blind people.

DEVELOPMENT AND DESCRIPTION OF THE METHODS USED IN THE SOFTWARE DEVELOPMENT PROCESS

As it has been mentioned, the user was involved from the first stage of software development using the card sorting and thinking aloud methods as indicated by the methodology proposed by Álvarez, t. (2018).

The thinking aloud method was implemented in the design and testing stages while the card sorting method was implemented in the design stage.

To carry out the evaluation of the methods, 5 blind people were considered. Álvarez, t. (2018) indicates based on Nielsen (2012) what, five is the number of people needed to perform exploratory tests to evaluate a modified method.

Description of the Used Methods

The methods that were used to evaluate usability and UX during the software development process correspond to Thinking Aloud and Card Sorting.

Thinking Aloud

In Thinking Aloud method the participants say what they are doing and thinking while completing a task, revealing aspects that they like or dislike. At the time of performing the evaluation is to be recorded to not lose any details.

Card Sorting

The Card Sorting method obtains information from where the users expect to have placed the components of the ISS, the user is given a series of printed cards, which the blind user classifies them in the order in which they prefer.

Description of Work Development by Stages of Development of the Software Cycle and Obtained Results

At each stage of software development, a method was applied with which results were obtained. Each of the results obtained allowed us to make modifications and continue with the development of the ISS.

Analysis Stage

In the Analysis stage no method proposed in the methodology was implemented, however, the requirements and needs of blind users were captured by interviews where information was collected about the desired application, with this we realized about mental perception and needs that the blind users had regarding the application.

Analysis Stage Results

Thanks to the information obtained during the interviews, the software development team identified the following functional and non-functional requirements for ISS of Braille, which were presented to the blind user and they were agreed on them. (see Table 1 and Table 2).

Table 1. Functional requirements

Key	Functional requirements
RF-01	The system has an introduction to train the user on navigation in the application.
RF-02	The system will randomly display an alphabet letter in Braille language for user learning.
RF-03	The system will test the user learning with alphabet exercises in Braille language which will appear randomly.
RF-04	The system will display random digits from zero to nine (0, 1, 2, 3, 4, 5, 6, 7.8 and 9) in Braille language for user learning.
RF-05	The system will test user learning with Braille digit exercises which will randomly appear from zero to nine (0, 1, 2, 3, 4, 5, 6, 7, 8, and 9).
RF-06	The system will randomly display an accented or unaccented vowel in Braille language for user learning.
RF-07	The system will test the user's learning with accented or non-accentuated vocal exercises in Braille language which will appear randomly.
RF-08	The system will randomly display the symbols comma (,), period (.), Colon (:), interrogation (?), Exclamation (!), Hyphen (-), underscore (_), at (@) and next capital letter symbol in braille language for user learning.
RF-09	The system will test the user learning with symbol exercises (comma (,), period (.), Colon (:), interrogation (?), Exclamation (!), Hyphen (-), underscore (_), at (@) and next capital letter) in Braille language which will appear randomly.
RF-10	The system will test the user though exercises of a random word made of 4 letters so that the user implements what has been learned in the application.

Source: Own Creation

Table 2. Non-functional requirements

Key	Non-functional requirements
RNF-01	The system will respond to the user's touch in less than 1 second.
RNF-02	The system will be able to respond quickly to N touch of the user.
RNF-03	The system will be responsive according to the device to be installed.
RNF-04	The system should provide hearing error messages that are informative.

Source: Own Creation

Design Stage

As mentioned, in the Design stage, Card Sorting and Thinking Aloud methods were used. At this stage, several proposals for software prototypes were given to the user according to the information gathered at the Analysis stage.

Design Stage Implementing Card Sorting Method

For Card Sorting method, the procedure described in Álvarez, T. (2018) was followed, in a way and for the purposes of this application, cards were made so that blind users could perform the test (see Figure 1), all this to evaluate the order of menu.

Five users with ages ranging from 27 to 41 years participated in the Card Sorting test. All users have basic knowledge in the use of a mobile device, this aspect is important since the ISS will be developed for mobile devices.

It was expected that the final result of each blind user it was similar to the one proposed below:

- **Menu 1**
  - Tutorial
    - Description of the screen
    - Explore the screen
    - Description of the menu
    - Submenu description
    - Practice
- **Menu 2**
  - Vowels
    - Learn the vowels
    - Practice the vowels

Figure 1. Category cards and assignments written in Braille
Source: Own creation

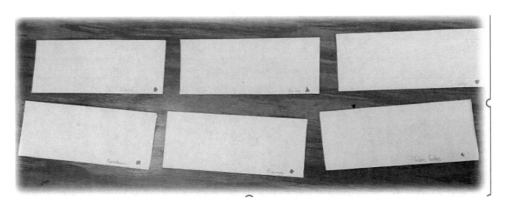

- **Menu 3**
  - ○ Numbers
    - ▪ Learn the numbers
    - ▪ Practice the numbers
- **Menu 4**
  - ○ Symbology
    - ▪ Learn the symbols
    - ▪ Practice the symbols
- **Menu 5**
  - ○ Alphabet
    - ▪ Learn the consonants
    - ▪ Practice the consonants
- **Menu 6**
  - ○ Short words
    - ▪ Learn to write

To carry out the Card Sorting procedure, each user was provided with 14 cards to be categorized and it was explained that there were 6 categories, they were ordering the cards in the category they considered appropriate. (see Figure 2 and Figure 3).

Results of the Design Stage With the Card Sorting Method

During the method evaluation some users made proposals on adding/modifying some task/category. Based on user feedback and method results, the following issues were changed:

Figure 2. Participant carrying out the test
Source: Own creation

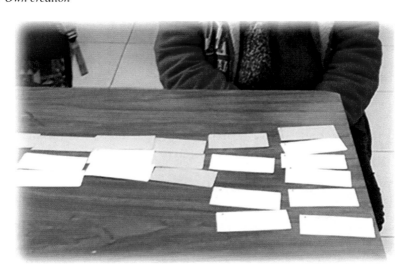

Figure 3. Result of the participant at the end of the method
Source: Own Creation

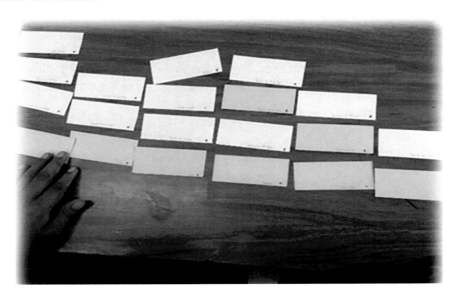

1. The name of the Alphabet category was modified to Consonants
2. The name of the Tutorial category was modified to Training
3. In the Tutorial category was removed the description screen option which was included in the option to Explore Screen
4. Homework learns to write modified to learn Short Words

Design Stage Implementing Thinking Aloud Method

For the method Thinking Aloud, the implemented procedure was the one described in Álvarez, T. (2018), where a tangible prototype based on reliefs was presented to the blind users, which was composed of 4 general system screens (see Figure 4). The users were exploring the prototype screens that were indicated and at the same time they shared their opinions about the prototype presented.

The software developers proposed 4 general screens in the system, which are made Spanish language. (see Figure 4). It should be noted that the system has more than 4 screens presented, but the ISS only has 4 screens with different structure, the only thing that varies is the name of the components and these names are changed according to what the user selected at the time of performing tasks in the application. The developers decided not to vary too much the structure of the screens so that the blind user quickly became familiar with the with the screens. Three of the four screens presented correspond to menus of the application, and only one to the blind user's workspace.

At the time of implemented the evaluation method Thinking Aloud, each user was provided for 4 screens with reliefs to identify the sections proposed for each screen,

Figure 4. Prototype screens
Source: Own creation

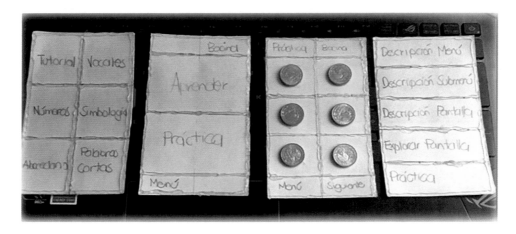

the blind user was guided to identify the location and name of the components in each proposed screen, at the same time the blind users were free to express what they thought about each of the screens (see Figure 5).

In general terms, the user expressed that he felt the application was adequate and only expressed a couple of modifications which are shown in the results section of the method.

Result of Design Stage With Thinking Aloud Method

In the Thinking Aloud method, opinions were obtained of what the user was thinking about when he went exploring the prototype presented of the ISS. Thanks to the opinions presented, the following changes were made:

1. In the main menu, the order of the proposed categories was modified, left to right: Tutorial, Vowels, Consonants, Numbers, Symbols and last Short Words (see Figure 6)
2. The Tutorial submenu screen was reduced to Scan Screen and Learn Functionality, so the Description Options Menu, Submenu Description and

Figure 5. User doing the method thinking aloud
Source: Own creation

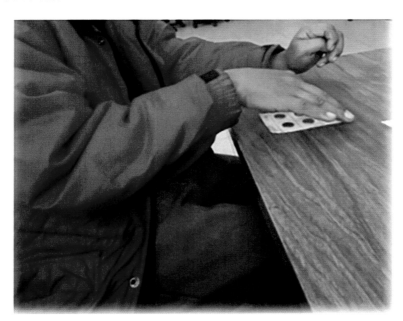

Practice were eliminated where its functionality was implemented in the option to Scan Screen (see Figure 7)

Design Stage Results

Thanks to the implementation of Thinking Aloud and Card Sorting methods, it was possible to gather information about the desired final structure in the ISS by blind users. With the methods we were able to identify the ideal order and name each component within the software.

The final interfaces based on the results are shown below: (see Figures 6,7,8,9 and 10).

In the development stage any method proposed in the methodology of Álvarez, T. (2018) was implemented., However, the development of the software was performed with the information obtained in the Design stage, in which as well mentioned were used Thinking Aloud and Card Sorting methods.

The Braille system was developed for mobile devices (MD), for this reason the programming language of Android was used, according to Barroso (2015) and the website Market statistics for Internet technologies (2018) indicate that Android is the language of most used programming for MD.

Figure 6. Main menu screen
Source: Own creation

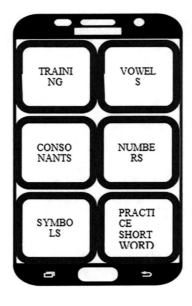

Figure 7. Screen of the tutorial submenu
Source: Own creation

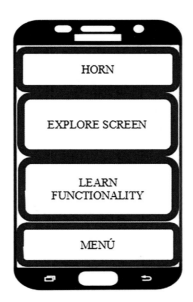

Figure 8. Work screen practice (writing)
Source: Own creation

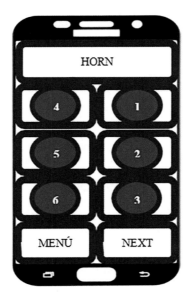

Figure 9. Work screen learn (reading)
Source: Own Creation

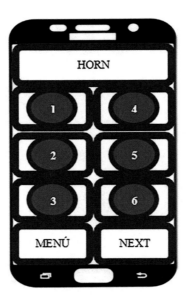

Figure 10. Screen of Submenu; x: can be vowels, consonants, numbers and symbols on two sections only in practice add short words
Source: Own Development Stage

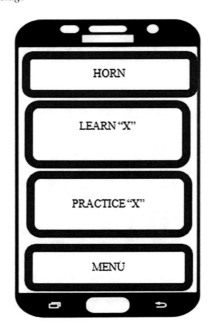

The integrated development environment (IDE) used was the Android Studio 3.1.2 software, and the application was developed for versions of Jelly bean 4.2 and up. since 94% of MDs use this version as a start stop (Barroso, 2015).

For the development of the software it was considered to support TalkBack as Herrero, G. (2013) indicates that it is an accessibility tool implemented by Android, which allows a blind person to use the mobile device with relative ease because it consists of informing by voice everything that happens on the phone's screen. So, it is important to consider that to use the ISS it is necessary to activate this option on the mobile device.

Development Stage Results

In the Development stage, the ISS was fully developed with the information obtained in the Design stage through their Card Sorting and Thinking Aloud methods. The final screens of the ISS are shown below (see Figures 11, 12, 13, 14, 15, y 16).

Figure 11. Main menu
Source: Own creation

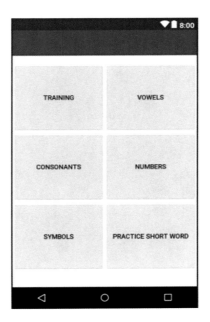

Figure 12. Short word screen
Source: Own creation

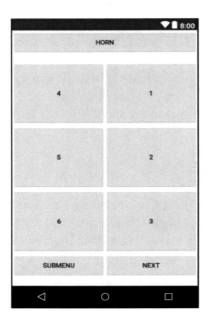

Figure 13. Submenu screen
Source: Own creation

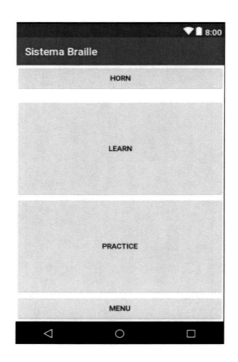

Figure 14. Work screen learn (reading)
Source: Own creation

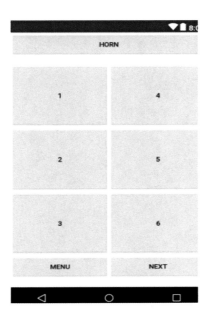

Figure 15. Training screen
Source: Own creation

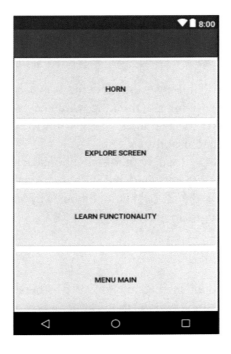

Figure 16. Work screen practice (writing)
Source: Own creation

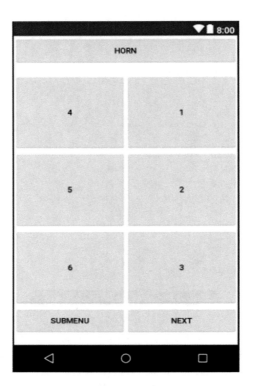

Testing Stage

In the Testing stage, the Thinking Aloud method was used in which 5 blind users verbalized what they were doing and thinking while they were completing a task in the ISS delivered, thanks to this method it was possible to evaluate the final software in accordance with UX and usability.

At the time of Thinking Aloud method evaluation, each user was provided with a mobile device with the ISS installed and with its respective activated TalkBack tool; the users were doing the tasks in autonomous way and at the same time they expressed what they thought about each screen.

Testing Stage Results

Thanks to the Thinking Aloud method implemented in this stage an improvement was identified, which will be implemented to the system, this improvement is localized in the learning task (see Figure 15) and corresponds to indicate through voice if the selected point is correct or incorrect; in spite of the information gathered in the previous stages where was established that when a user touches one of the braille buttons and this is was correct, the mobile only vibrated and if it is not correct, it does not do anything; the users indicated that he seemed more comfortable the new form indicated for such reason this improvement will be made in the future.

CONCLUSION

It is possible to conclude that, to achieve a usable application focused on a person with some type of disability, in this case blind users, it is essential to rely on a methodology that allows to evaluate the usability and allows us to involve both the user and the experts in development and as a result a satisfied customer is expected since the software covers the requirements and expectations of this.

It is considered very important that the user has had power to decision from the early stages of development system as this facilitated generating proposals for the product desirable by the user, for this reason it is considered that the Thinking Aloud and Card Sorting methods proposed by Álvarez, T. (2018) are efficient to achieve usability and satisfactory UX because they involve the user since the beginning of development process.

The Álvarez, T. (2018) methodology performs appropriate usability evaluations and thanks to this development is considered to be upper than the existing methodologies, as indicated in work of Álvarez, T. (2018) than the authors (Virtanen, 2003), (Kulyukin y cols., 2004) that there is software that has been developed for the blind people but they don't consider adequate usability evaluations.

REFERENCES

Aguilera Hintelholher, R. (2013). Identidad y diferenciación entre Método y Metodología. *Estudios Politicos*, *9*(28), 81–103. doi:10.1016/S0185-1616(13)71440-9

Álvarez, T. (2018). *Metodología para la evaluación de la experiencia del usuario en sistemas de software interactivos para usuarios ciegos (Tesis de doctorado)*. Universidad Veracruzana.

Arhippainen, L. (2003). *Capturing user experience for product design*. IRIS26, the 26th Information Systems Research Seminar in Scandinavia, Porvoo, Finland. Retrieved from = http://www.vtt.fi/virtual/adamos/material/arhippa2.pdf

Arhippainen, L., & Tähti, M. (2003). Empirical Evaluation of User Experience in Two Adaptative Mobile Application Prototypes. *Proceedings of the 2nd International Conference on Mobile and Ubiquitous Multimedia*. Retrieved from http://www.ep.liu.se/ecp/011/007/ecp011007.pdf

Barroso, A. (2015). *Aplicación Android para un recorrido monumental virtual por Segovia (Tesis de grado)*. Universidad de Valladolid.

Granollers, T., Lorés, V., Sendin, M., & Perdrix, F. (2005). Integración de la ipo y la ingeniería del software: Mpiu+. *Taller en Sistemas Hipermedia Colaborativos y Adaptativos*, 25.

Herrero, G. (2013). *Ayuda para invidentes utilizando teléfonos Android (Tesis de grado)*. Universidad Autónoma de Madrid.

Kulyukin, V., Gharpure, C., Nicholson, J., & Pavithran, S. (2004). Rd in robot-assisted indoor navigation for the visually impaired. In Intelligent robots and systems, 2004. (iros 2004). proceedings. 2004 ieee/rsj international conference on (Vol. 2, pp. 1979-1984). Academic Press.

Mioduser, D., & Lahav, O. (2004). Anticipatory cognitive mapping of unknown spaces by people who are blind using a virtual learning environment. In *Proceedings of the 6th international conference on learning sciences* (pp. 334-341). Academic Press.

Nielsen, J. (2012). *Nielsen-norman group - evidence-based user experience research, training and consulting*. Retrieved from http://www.nngroup.com/articles/how-many-test-users/

Nielsen, J., & Loranger, H. (2006). *Usabilidad. Prioridad en el diseño web*. Madrid: Anaya.

Operating System Market Share. (2018). *Market Share Statistics for Internet Technologies website*. Retrieved from https://www.netmarketshare.com

Pérez, J. P., & Gardey, A. (2008). *Definición de método*. Retrieved from https://definicion.de/metodo/

Sánchez, J. (2010). Una metodología para desarrollar y evaluar la usabilidad de entornos virtuales basados en audio para el aprendizaje y la cognición de usuarios ciegos [A methodology for developing and evaluating the usability of audio-based virtual environments for learning and cognition of blind people]. *Revista Iberoamericana de Educación a Distancia*, *13*(2), 265.

Sánchez, J., Tadres, A., Pascual-Leone, A., & Merabet, L. (2009). Blind children navigation through gaming and associated brain plasticity. In 2009 virtual rehabilitation international conference (pp. 29-36). Academic Press. doi:10.1109/ICVR.2009.5174201

Virtanen, A. (2003). Navigation and guidance system for the blind. *Proceedings of Interactive Future and Man, 1.*

Chapter 8

Use of Audio–Based Mobile Assistant for Reading Texts as Support for Blind Users

Alfonso Sánchez Orea
Universidad Veracruzana, Mexico

ABSTRACT

In order to give visually impaired people a greater degree of inclusion in society, it is necessary to consider not only aspects related to independence in their physical mobility but also in their intellectual and labor mobility. Currently if a blind person needs information from a book, it must be previously translated in Braille language; in addition, the person must know this language or in the absence there should be the audio version. Most public and private libraries do not currently have books in Braille versions or in their absence audio books, so getting the information to perform some task is complicated. On the other hand, translating books from their original version into Braille language or its audio version is a titanic and expensive task, so in the chapter, the authors propose a technological solution based on the mobile platforms for the blind to perform this task in the place and time necessary without more resources than a Smartphone.

DOI: 10.4018/978-1-5225-8539-8.ch008

INTRODUCTION

We have all heard different terms used to refer to people with visual disabilities, often not knowing the officially accepted terms or their definition. In the International Classification of Functioning, Disability and Health (World Health Organization), disability is considered as "a generic term that includes deficits, limitations in activity and restrictions on participation" (2018).

For the INEGI, disability is a term that "includes the deficiencies in the structures and functions of the human body, the limitations in the personal capacity to carry out basic tasks of daily life and the restrictions in the social participation that the individual experiences" ("General Law", 2013).

In Mexico, in May 2011 the General Law for the Inclusion of Persons with Disabilities was published in the Official Gazette of the Federation, establishing the conditions under which the State should promote, protect and ensure the full exercise of human rights and rights. Fundamental freedoms of people with disabilities, ensuring their full inclusion in society in a framework of respect, equality and equalization of opportunities. This law recognizes their human rights and mandates the establishment of the necessary public policies for their exercise ("General Law").

According to the INEGI in 2010, for every 100 people with disabilities, 27 reported having difficulty seeing, even wearing glasses, which represents around 1.6 million individuals in the country, a number only exceeded by those with mobility limitations; that is to say, the visual limitations occupy second place in the country (INEGL, 2013).

The "Digital gap" is the distance that exists in the different activities of individuals and their geographical, social or work environments in the different socioeconomic strata in relation to their opportunities to access ICT and Internet use (INEGL, 2013). One of the most vulnerable populations in this context are people with some disability, because they do not have the availability of information, access to education or public spaces. The educational institutions, governmental and private, operate without thinking about all the capacities of the population that inhabits them. Get the displacement from one place to another for a person with visual impairment (DV) in the city or town where they live so they can perform their daily activities such as going to work, school, supermarket or perform a procedure of any kind it can be a complex activity. Most people with DV perform these tasks in the company of a family member and very rarely do it independently (OECD, 2001).

If a person with a visual disability has access to sources of information in an appropriate format, it can increase their intellectual, social and work development, facilitating the solution of some problems in their environment and thus improve their economic conditions (OECD, 2001).

Even though there are laws that protect people with visual disabilities from discrimination, they are still part of the most vulnerable population to suffer it. Having easy access to information, education, health or public spaces has always been a difficult challenge for them to overcome. The educational and governmental institutions have initiated the implementation of measures that help this inclusion, these measures range from awareness programs, modification of physical spaces, printing of texts in major typology to technological proposals for mobility in open and closed spaces ("Children's Day", 2013).

The ability to use ICT is characterized by the ability to receive, manipulate and process information immediately, in different formats and in a variety of mobile or fixed devices. Modern society is becoming more expert in the use of ICTs, increasing the degree of polarization of ICTs; At one extreme are the people who handle ICT in their personal and work life, focused on expanding their professional development through the opportunity of access to information sources in order to improve their academic development, communicate through knowledge networks and solve problems of their environment, on the other point are those who do not have access to these resources, resulting in inequalities, exclusions and social struggles ("Children's Day", 2013).

THEORETICAL FRAMEWORK

According to the World Health Organization, the visual function is divided into four levels: - Normal vision. - Moderate visual impairment (low vision). - Severe visual impairment (low vision). - Blindness. This work will focus mainly on the sector with blindness, but without leaving aside people with low vision (World Health Organization, 2018).

The guide "Inclusive Education. People with Visual Disability ", elaborated in the Institute of Educational Technologies (ITE) of Spain, mentions some of the complications that occur in People with Visual Disabilities, among which the following stand out ("Children's Day", 2013).

- Difficulty in receiving information from the environment. - By requiring, generally, the combined use of the other senses, it may take the person more time to receive certain information.

- Difficulty learning by imitation.
- Use of verbalisms or echolalia.
- Possible scattered attention.
- Deficiency of non-verbal social skills (such as facial expressions).

To combat the above obstacles, the guide suggests some points that should be worked with the People with Visual Disability (Frutos, 2012).

- Learning adaptive behaviors (and non-verbal social behaviors).
- Auditory stimulation (both for academic learning and to know elements present in their environment).
- Stimulation of the sense of taste and smell (identify and discriminate olfactory and gustatory sensations).
- Psychomotor stimulation.
- Adjustment of learning rhythms (avoiding their exclusion from a group).
- Specific programs of orientation and mobility techniques (to increase their autonomy and self-esteem).
- Adaptation of the environment to the educational and social needs of the student (location of the student in the classroom, optical and non-optical aids, among others). Assigning a specific space, close to the teacher, allows the student to reach his or her place independently and feel confident of having the teacher close to him.

It should be mentioned that the person with visual disability "does not develop the other senses" necessarily, this is achieved by the need that is presented and the practice of using them, which is essential for an adequate academic development. Each sense generates in a person mental and sensory images. Although the most used by people without visual disabilities are precisely those created by that sense, this shows us that People with Visual Disability can occupy the images constructed by the rest of the senses.

The ITE guide points out that the student with visual impairment must process auditory information by (Frutos, 2012).

- Attention. Determine that there is a sound.
- Identification. Recognize what sound you are listening to.
- Discrimination. Distinguish one sound from another.
- Location. Identify the origin of a sound.
- Tracking. Move to the source of a sound.

According to the INEGI (See, Figure 1), the level of education of a person corresponds to the highest cycle of studies reached by the population of 3 years and more in the levels of the National Education System, these levels are: basic, upper and higher. Among the population with limitations to see, of every 100 people of 15 years and over, 25 did not complete any degree of the National Educational System, 60 finished at least one grade of the basic level, 8 at least some of the upper middle and 6 one of the superior (INEGL, 2013).

In Mexico, for almost 50 years primary textbooks have been published in Braille by the National Commission of Free Textbooks (CONALITEG), in 2013, began the publication of books in macro types (large letters) for Weak visuals and from the beginning of this school year textbooks for secondary in Braille were published for the first time ("Children's Day", 2013). CONALITEG despite having its own printing machines to make books in Braille, for 2014 it had to rely on independent printers to produce 20% of what it needed for the current school year. Editing a book in Braille costs up to 40% more than those printed in ink (Diaz, 2015).

The "José Vasconcelos" library in the Federal District has a Braille room where reading aloud services, Braille printing, text readers, loan of equipment with speaking voice, 400 titles of audio books, enlarging machines text and a Braille collection of 500 titles (Diaz, 2015). In the National Library of the UNAM, of University City in its room of Tiflológico they are counted on 1,799 titles of 474 authors in Braille, reading and automated recording, edition of printed materials (programs Screen Reader, Open Book and Jaws), amplification of characters, transcription of

Figure 1. Percentage distribution of the population aged 15 and over, by sex according to level of education, Source: INEGI. 2010 Population and Housing Census. Note: The unspecified for each level of schooling is not presented: total (0.8%), men (0.8%) and women (0.7%).

Level of education	Total	Mens	Women
Total	100	100	100
None	25.00	20.80	28.80
Basic level	59.70	61.60	58.00
Medium superior level	8.30	9.20	7.40
Upper level	6.20	7.60	5.00

Braille to common characters and vice versa, as well as training workshops in the management of equipment ("Bibliotheca Central", 2018).

Although government efforts have been made, there is no institutional policy that brings Mexicans with visual impairment closer to literature or knowledge. When a material in Braille is needed that does not exist, it usually requests its transcription to any of the existing civil organizations or the La Salle University that dedicate themselves to it, they have catalogs of books that they have transcribed on their own initiative (IAP, 2013).

In Mexico, there is no school that trains Braille text transcribers, this can be a major problem, because it is necessary to know the cognitive process of a blind person and adapt the text to their understanding of the world, that the blind or visually impaired do not want to use Braille because they consider it boring and complex, so they prefer to use audiobooks (INTEF, 2019).

If it is intended to achieve greater inclusion of people with visual impairment in access to reading and knowledge contained in books to achieve greater schooling that allows you to increase your intellectual, social, work and economic development should seek new alternatives. One of these is the incorporation of mobile technological solutions in the transcription of audio texts ("Lanacion", 2019).

One of the biggest challenges in the development of technological tools for people with visual disabilities, is that they are accepted and mainly used by these users, therefore we must create user-friendly interfaces under the principles of User-Centered Design to ensure that the application has the appropriate functionality for the needs and capabilities of specific users. In this particular case of people with visual impairments audio-based interfaces are needed because they use the sense of hearing as the main source of awareness.

The User-Centered Design (DCU) (Human-centered design) is described according to the ISO 13407 standard (Vargas, 2011).

Human-centered design is characterized by: the active involvement of users and a clear understanding of user and task requirements; an appropriate allocation of function between users and technology; the iteration of design solutions; multi-disciplinary design.

His concept includes involving the user and understanding their needs so that technological solutions can be implemented according to these requirements. The standard also proposes to divide the User-Centered Design process into four phases (Hassan-Montero, Y.; Ortega-Santamaría, S.; 2009) (See Figure 2)

Figure 2. Design process focused on the user

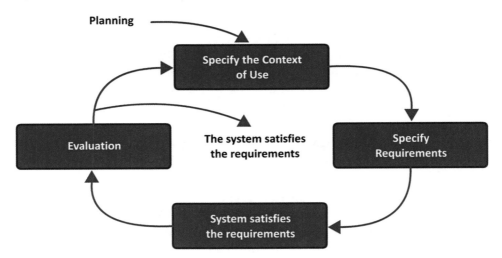

- Understand and specify the context of use: Identify the people to whom the product is directed, for what they will use it and under what conditions.
- **Specify Requirements:** Identify the objectives of the user and the supplier of the product should be satisfied.
- **Produce Design Solutions:** This phase can be subdivided into different sequential stages, from the first conceptual solutions to the final design solution.
- **Evaluation:** It is the most important phase of the process, in which the design solutions are validated (the system satisfies the requirements) or, on the contrary, usability problems are detected, usually through user tests.

Some authors divide the User-Centered Design into only three main stages, encompassing the first two stages of the previous classification into one:

- Know the end users thoroughly.
- Design a product that fits your abilities, motivations and expectations and solve your needs.
- Test the designed product.

The "User Test" mentioned aims to answer the questions:

- **What?:** The main points that will be tested by users.
- **How?:** The way in which they will be tested (what tools will be needed, for example).
- **When?:** The tests must be carried out during the development process to detect errors or possible improvements in time and reduce the probability of generating costly corrections (in time, money and effort) at the end.

Currently there are a lot of tools that facilitate access to information, for example, a computer, one of the most important is the screen reader. A screen reader tries to identify and interpret what is displayed on a computer screen to represent it alternatively, usually by voice or with a braille line. It belongs to the group of tools called assistive technology that facilitates or allows people with disabilities to perform some types of tasks. The most popular screen readers employ a speech synthesizer, which is a system capable of artificially producing human speech (Vargas, 2011).

Among the most used desktop screen reader's stand out two: JAWS and NVDA. Some of the main differences between the two are:

- JAWS works exclusively on Windows operating systems. While this makes it less portable, it also provides greater speed in accessing system resources more directly. NVDA can be used in various operating systems.
- NVDA sometimes does not read all the elements of web pages (JAWS usually read almost all), however, NVDA can read some Flash elements.
- JAWS allows, in general, to navigate in a more user-friendly manner through Microsoft Office package software, however, NVDA better addresses a variety of different programs, such as the calculator.
- Being open source NVDA, the community can create add-ons ("add-ons") to add functions, and the user can download them as soon as they are released. To obtain a new functionality in JAWS, you must wait for it to be implemented by the developers of the program itself, and then buy it together with a new version.

In 2015, Google introduced a feature that allows instant text translation through a smartphone camera, translating it into 36 different languages. It also incorporates a conversation mode that uses Google's voice command and cloud storage to translate the dialogue between two people who speak different languages. This new function can help sectors with important roles in the growing multicultural communities such as people with visual disabilities (Mountero et al, 2019).

METHODOLOGY

Before explaining the methodology, a diagram is presented that explains in a general way the operation of the developed application. See Figure 3.

If you want to develop an application for a mobile device regardless of its platform or its environment, it is necessary to recognize and establish the conditions that guarantee the relevance, quality, security, efficiency and performance of the application that you want to build and use medium of the mobile device. It is important to follow the general stages of the software life cycle, considering the differences that exist between the development of an application to run on a desktop PC and that of an application to run on a mobile device.

This proposal of development methodology is composed of the stages of the life cycle of software for mobile devices added with a stage of Usability Testing. See Figure 4.

1. Definition of requirements: The specification of the requirements of the users is defined, which in this case are users with visual disability; the problem to be addressed, the reading of texts that are not written in Braille, and whether the application justifies a mobile development.

Figure 3. General outline of the operation of the Mobile Assistant to translate text into audio

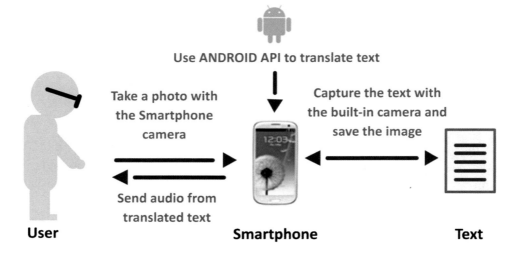

Figure 4. Life cycle of software development for applications in mobile devices adding a stage of Usability Testing.

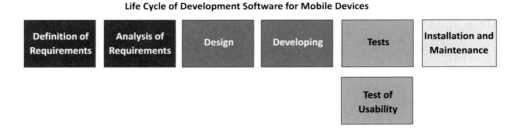

2.   Analysis of requirements: The entries that will be the written texts, the processes, and the outputs are identified and represented, which is the audio result of the translation of texts and the users that intervene directly in the mobile application, which has already mentioned are people with visual disabilities.

3.   Design: The visual and technical aspects that give life to the mobile application are defined very clearly, feedback is generated by the user, functional aspects are defined with the user regarding navigability, movements through the device and the way of loading, storage and presentation of the data requested and necessary for the process required by the mobile application. To emulate the user interfaces in the design you must use mobile device emulators.

4.   Development: In this stage the source code that allows the operation of the mobile software is written, the programming language is defined, which in this case is ANDROID and the APIs for text translation and conversion to audio format. This language used for mobile programming must be adapted to the design needs previously agreed with the direct users of the application.

5.   Testing: At this stage, it must be verified that the software complies with the requirements defined in previous stages and generates the results expected by the users.

   a.   **Unit Tests:** When building a mobile application, it is vital to check that the written source code works correctly and adapts to the permanent operation of the program.

   b.   **Integration Tests:** Not only the individual functioning of the mobile software must be tested, but also its integration with the other components of the application, especially with the data server with which the synchronization process of the information used in the device.

   c.   **Validation Tests:** This process aims to determine if the mobile application meets the objectives for which the product was built.

In this stage, a section of Usability Testing was added, which allows knowing precisely if the application meets the real needs of the type of user for whom it was developed, in this case, if the interface is usable for people with visual disabilities. Three different test moments were defined:

1.   **Initial.** Handling the Smartphone, touch tests and audio tests.
2.   **Medium.** Use of the audio interface of the application, understanding of the initial instructions, text capture, handling of the distances of the Smartphone with respect to the text.
3.   **Final.** Use of the interface with the camera, understanding of audio indications, storage of text for consultation.

At the end of each test period, an oral survey was conducted to the users to know to what degree the application is accepted and thus be able to make the necessary modifications to obtain an acceptable degree of usability.

The purpose of the questionnaire that follows is to evaluate the functionalities of the application prototype "Use of audio-based mobile assistant for reading texts as support for blind users". The information provided by the participants is confidential, ensuring that no other use will be given to their answers other than to evaluate the usability degree of this prototype.

Personal Information

Age: _____
Gender: _____

Maximum degree of Schooling: _____

1.   How much have you used a Smartphone?
     a.   More than 20 times
     b.   More than 5 times
     c.   One time
     d.   Never
2.   Why do you use the Smartphone more often?
     a.   Make calls
     b.   Listen to music
     c.   Location Application
     d.   Other: _____

3. Have you used the Talkback accessibility option for Visual Disability of your Smartphone?
    a. yes
    b. no
4. In the affirmative case of the previous question. In what degree has it been useful to perform some function of your Smartphone?
    a. Large extent
    b. Fair extent
    c. Barely
    d. Not at all
5. The voice that the Talkback uses to describe the interface of your Smartphone by default. How satisfying and useful do you think?
    a. Large extent
    b. Fair extent
    c. Barely
    d. Not at all
6. Are the voice instructions provided by the application easy to understand and follow?
    a. Large extent
    b. Fair extent
    c. Barely
    d. Not at all
7. After 5 sessions with the application. How difficult was it to follow the instructions to use the camera and calculate the focus distance of the text?
    a. Very difficult
    b. Difficult
    c. Something difficult
    d. Nothing difficult
8. After performing 5 test sessions with the application. How difficult was it to get the text of a page?
    a. Very difficult
    b. Difficult
    c. Something difficult
    d. Nothing difficult
9. To what degree do you consider that the audio that describes the captured text is understandable?
    a. Very understandable.
    b. Understandable.
    c. Little understandable.
    d. Nothing understandable.

10. After performing 5 test sessions with the application. How hard was it to get a page saved for later reference?
    a. Very difficult
    b. Difficult
    c. Something difficult
    d. Nothing difficult
11. From 1 to 10 considering that 1 is nothing and that 10 is very good. To what extent do you consider that this application fulfills the function of translating written text to audio for its understanding?
    a. 1-3
    b. 3-5
    c. 5-8
    d. 9-10

RESULTS

The first prototype of the mobile assistant was developed, which allows reading textbooks and converting them into audio at the image capture site. See Figure 5.

In this first version you can store up to 3 pages in the memory of the device for later reading by means of audio and it is possible to translate at least 20 different types of sources, it was installed in a LG80 Smartphone, with 4GB of storage, with 8 megapixel camera with Android 4.2 Operating System.

Figure 5. Prototype tests of the audio-based mobile assistant for reading texts to support people with visual impairments

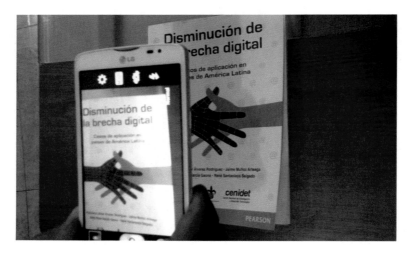

The pilot usability tests were conducted on 6 people with visual disabilities who attend the Sala Braille of the School Normal Veracruzana in the city of Xalapa, Veracruz

Main characteristics of the people with whom the application will be tested are described below in Figure 6. (Personal data are omitted for reasons of protection of your data).

After 5 sessions of pilot tests the evaluation instrument was applied and the results are shown in Figures 7-17.

Figure 6. Main characteristics of blind people in which the application will be tested

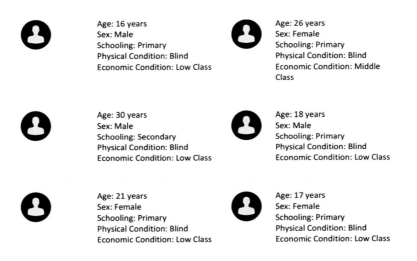

Age: 16 years
Sex: Male
Schooling: Primary
Physical Condition: Blind
Economic Condition: Low Class

Age: 26 years
Sex: Female
Schooling: Primary
Physical Condition: Blind
Economic Condition: Middle Class

Age: 30 years
Sex: Male
Schooling: Secondary
Physical Condition: Blind
Economic Condition: Low Class

Age: 18 years
Sex: Male
Schooling: Primary
Physical Condition: Blind
Economic Condition: Low Class

Age: 21 years
Sex: Female
Schooling: Primary
Physical Condition: Blind
Economic Condition: Low Class

Age: 17 years
Sex: Female
Schooling: Primary
Physical Condition: Blind
Economic Condition: Low Class

Figure 7. Results of question: How much have you used a Smartphone?

1. HOW MUCH HAVE YOU USED A SMARTPHONE?

■ a)   More than 20 times   ■ b)   More than 5 times

■ c)   One time   ■ d)   Never

0%
17%
50%
33%

Figure 8. Results of question: Why do you use the Smartphone more often?

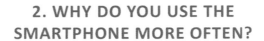

2. WHY DO YOU USE THE SMARTPHONE MORE OFTEN?

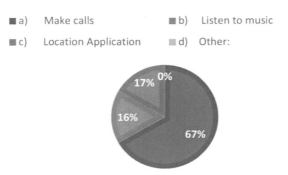

Figure 9. Results of question: Have you used the Talkback accessibility option for Visual Disability of your Smartphone?

3. HAVE YOU USED THE TALKBACK ACCESSIBILITY OPTION FOR VISUAL DISABILITY OF YOUR SMARTPHONE?

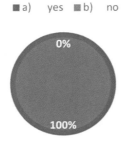

Despite being a pilot usability test in which only 6 blind people participate, it is important to highlight that all the people who participated in this test had already used a Smartphone more than 5 times and that they have used it for various applications. To make phone calls. 100% of the participants have used the accessibility tools provided by their Smarthphone and have been able to use it with some ease, being of their liking at a high level.

Figure 10. Results of question: In what degree has it been useful to perform some function of your Smartphone?

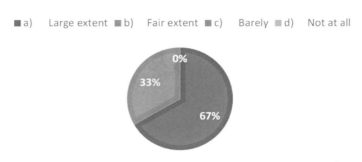

Figure 11. Results of question: The voice that the Talkback uses to describe the interface of your Smartphone by default. How satisfying and useful do you think?

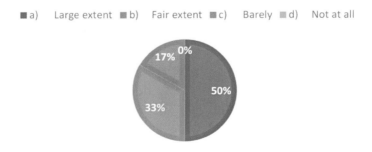

Regarding the use of the prototype, 89% consider that the application is easy to use and understand, although it requires more training and sessions of use, but in a considerably acceptable percentage most of the participants managed to follow the instructions, take the photograph, capture the text, translate it and store the result.

Figure 12. Results of question: Are the voice instructions provided by the application easy to understand and follow?

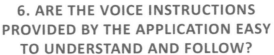

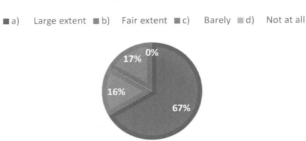

Figure 13. Results of question: How difficult was it to follow the instructions to use the camera and calculate the focus distance of the text?

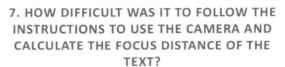

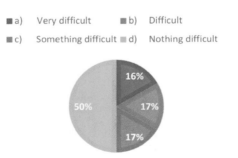

CONCLUSION

As this newly created application and one of the first efforts to support people with visual impairment in reading books that are not in Braille, a niche of opportunity for the development of applications that include other different types of Smartphone as well as other operating systems and programming languages. The importance

Figure 14. Results of question: How difficult was it to get the text of a page?

8. HOW DIFFICULT WAS IT TO GET THE TEXT OF A PAGE?

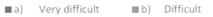

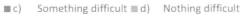

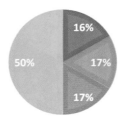

Figure 15. Results of question: To what degree do you consider that the audio that describes the captured text is understandable?

9. TO WHAT DEGREE DO YOU CONSIDER THAT THE AUDIO THAT DESCRIBES THE CAPTURED TEXT IS UNDERSTANDABLE?

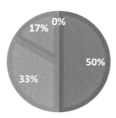

of the usability tests as part of the user-centered design to correct and adapt the application to the user's needs and abilities was highlighted.

Although it was developed for users with this disability, it can also be used by people who cannot read and who need to know textbook information in an audio format. Our goal is to design and develop a functional prototype in a low-cost

Figure 16. Results of question: How hard was it to get a page saved for later reference?

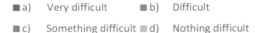

10 .HOW HARD WAS IT TO GET A PAGE SAVED FOR LATER REFERENCE?

■ a)   Very difficult   ■ b)   Difficult

■ c)   Something difficult ■ d)   Nothing difficult

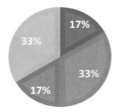

Figure 17. Results of question: To what extent do you consider that this application fulfills the function of translating written text to audio for its understanding?

11. TO WHAT EXTENT DO YOU CONSIDER THAT THIS APPLICATION FULFILLS THE FUNCTION OF TRANSLATING WRITTEN TEXT TO AUDIO FOR ITS UNDERSTANDING?

■ a)   1-3   ■ b)   3-5   ■ c)   5-8   ■ d)   9-10

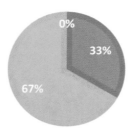

Smartphone with few capabilities, apply usability tests to a greater number of users with visual disabilities to obtain better results and perfect the OCR library that translates the text so that it can recognize different types of sources and other languages such as English.

REFERENCES

Bibliotecacentral.unam.mx. (2019). *Biblioteca Central*. Available at: http://bibliotecacentral.unam.mx/servdiscap.html

Díaz, V. (2015). Books in Braille, few and expensive. *MILENIO*. Available at: http://www.milenio.com/cultura/Libros-braille-pocos-caros_0_457154296.html

General Law for the Inclusion of Persons with Disabilities. (2013). *Official Gazette of the Federation*. Available at: http://www.diputados.gob.mx/LeyesBiblio/pdf/LGIPD.pdf

Hassan Montero, Y., & Ortega Santamaría, S. (2019). *APEI report on usability*. Available at: http://www.nosolousabilidad.com/manual/3.htm

IAP. (2013). *Association of the Visually Impaired IAP*. Available at: http://www.dis-capacidad.com/index.php

INEGI. (2013). *People with Disabilities in Mexico, a vision in 2010*. Available at: http://www.inegi.org.mx/prod_serv/contenidos/espanol/bvinegi/productos/censos/poblacion/2010/discapacidad/702825051785.pdf

INTEF. (2019). *Home - INTEF*. Available at: http://www.ite.educacion.es/formacion/materiales/129/cd/unidad_2/mo2_resumen

Lafuente de Frutos, Á. (2012). Inclusive education. People with Visual Disability Institute of Educational Technologies. Ministry of Education, Culture and Sports. Spain. National Commission of Free Textbooks (CONALITEG).

Lanacion.com.ar. (2019). *Google presentó una función que permite traducir texto con la cámara del teléfono*. Available at: http://www.lanacion.com.ar/1760090-google-presento-una-funcion-que-permite-traducir-mediante-la-camara-de-un-telefono-movil

Library, J. (2015). *José Vasconcelos Library*. SEP (Secretary of Public Education). Available at: http://www.bibliotecavasconcelos.gob.mx/espacios/braile/

OECD. (2001). *Understanding the Digital Divide*. Available at: http://www.oecd.org/dataoecd/38/57/1888451.pdf

On Children's Day, for Inclusive Education: respect for people with disabilities and indigenous population. (2013). Available at: http://www.conapred.org.mx/Documentos_cedoc / Dossier_Ed_Inclusiva_25_abril_2013_INACCSS.pdf

Vargas Agudelo, F. (2011). *Software Engineering in the development of applications for mobile devices* (1st ed.). Antioquia: TDA.

Vygotsky. (1997). *Lev Semenovitch. Selected Works V - Foundations of defectology. Translation: Julio Guillermo Blank*. Madrid: Viewer.

World Health Organization. (2018). *Blindness and visual impairment*. Available at: https://www.who.int/es/news-room/fact-sheets/detail/blindness-and-visual-impairment

Section 3
Working With Colorblind People

Chapter 9
Real–Time Recoloring Ishihara Plates Using Artificial Neural Networks for Helping Colorblind People

Martín Montes Rivera
(iD) https://orcid.org/0000-0003-3897-6212
Universidad Politécnica de Aguascalientes, Mexico

Juana Canul-Reich
(iD) https://orcid.org/0000-0003-1893-1332
Universidad Juárez Autónoma de Tabasco, Mexico

Alejandro Padilla
Universidad Autónoma de Aguascalientes, Mexico

Julio Ponce
Universidad Autónoma de Aguascalientes, Mexico

ABSTRACT

Vision sense is achieved using cells called rods (luminosity) and cones (color). Color perception is required when interacting with educational materials, industrial environments, traffic signals, among others, but colorblind people have difficulties perceiving colors. There are different tests for colorblindness like Ishihara plates test, which have numbers with colors that are confused with colorblindness. Advances in computer sciences produced digital assistants for colorblindness, but there are possibilities to improve them using artificial intelligence because its techniques have exhibited great results when classifying parameters. This chapter proposes the use of artificial neural networks, an artificial intelligence technique, for learning the colors that colorblind people cannot distinguish well by using as input data the Ishihara plates and recoloring the image by increasing its brightness. Results are tested with a real colorblind people who successfully pass the Ishihara test.

DOI: 10.4018/978-1-5225-8539-8.ch009

INTRODUCTION

The sense of sight allows biological organisms to acquire images of their environment, allowing them to identify food and dangers. Humans require its vision sense to read, write, identify signposts, drive, among other activities (Porrero & Juan M., 2005).

Vision is possible thanks to the eyes, which use two types of cells for the perception of images, the rods and the cones. (Richmond Products, 2016). The rods are sensitive to the amount of light or brightness perceived, i.e. the magnitude of the light wave. (Ruki Harwahyu, 2011). Light wave frequency or color is perceived through the cones, these cells are generally found in three variants that identify basic colors, i.e. the amount of red, green and blue perceived (Colblindor, 2016).

Color is a sense, which is in the brain and is obtained from the signals of the neurons connected to the cone outputs that are activated when light strikes the frequency corresponding to each photo receptor (Tanaka, 2015).

Usually people have only cones that perceive the red, green and blue colors and the other colors are obtained as the result of combinations that are generated by the interaction of light magnitudes in tune with the frequencies of these basic colors. (Deeb, 2004).

There are peculiar cases in which human beings have a fourth cone, as well as some species of birds, that is, they are tetrachromats, allowing them to perceive a greater range of colors, compared to the colors perceived by people who have three cones or trichromats (Tanaka, 2015; Robson, 2016).

Tetrachromats, despite having extrasensory abilities compared to most people, often have difficulty interacting with the world and expressing their opinions about some colors, as the environment is designed for trichromats which are dominant compared to other groups (Robson, 2016).

Colorblindness

There are also people who can perceive fewer colors than the average, this condition is called colorblindness, described in a scientific work for the first time in 1793 by John Dalton who also suffered from colorblindness, in his work it is mentioned that the perception of color is due to a colored liquid in the eyes, however, it is proven that this statement was not correct at the time of his death, when scientist analyze his eyes (Colblindor, 2016).

People with color blindness often have problems with their environment and the world in which they live, since as tetrachromats, have difficulties interacting with trichromats in activities that involve a correct perception of color. Some examples of these are: recreational activities with board games, discussion about objects and their identification, interpretation of signs or signals while driving, educational activities with colored material, among others. Such difficulties make color blindness a medium disability (Colblindor, 2016; Chieko Kato, 2013).

The frame of reference that defines the difficulties that a person with color blindness faces in his life can be very extensive, can affect the career that they choose, the positions and responsibilities assigned in their jobs, the choice of clothes they wear, the food they cook, the sports they play and even the simple fact of finding a parking space could be difficult (Antonio Tagarelli, 2004). Colorblindness in most cases is congenital due to genetic inheritance, however, it can be acquired by disease, stroke or infection that damages the photo-receptors of color, also some medications can cause temporary color blindness (Richmond Products, 2016; Colblindor, 2016; Deeb, 2004).

Variants of Color Blindness

Color blindness can be classified according to the cone with problems and how severe they are. In the first instance, color blindness is classified according to its severity into: anomalous trichromacy, dichromacy, monochromacy (Colblindor, 2016; Chieko Kato, 2013).

Anomalous trichromacy is the condition of greater prevalence, but of lesser severity and characterizes the people who can perceive tonalities with the red, green and blue cones, but they have deficiencies in some cones, which decreases its capability for perceiving the spectrum of colors reducing the amount of tonalities that can be identified (Hatem M. Marey, 2015). Anomalous trichromacy is divided into: protanomaly if there are difficulties in the perception of reds, deuteranomaly for problems with the perception of greens and tritanomaly if it is difficult to perceive tones with the blue cone (Chieko Kato, 2013).

When color blindness occurs with a specific absent cone, it is called dichromacy. In this variant, the colors generated with combinations of the absent cone cannot be perceived and this causes a severe difficulty identifying or perceiving colors (Chieko Kato, 2013). Dichromacy is subdivided according to the absent cone into: protanopia if you cannot perceive colors with the red cone, deuteranopia if you cannot see colors with the green tonality and tritanopia if the blue cone is absent (Hatem M. Marey, 2015).

When the perception of color is lost, the environment is perceived in grayscale or with variations of brightness, this condition is called monochromacy and is the most severe variant of colorblindness, but its occurrence is the lowest (Chieko Kato, 2013).

Colorblindness Perception

Awareness of people about colorblindness it is important because it is middle disability, for this reason, in recent years have been applied digital media, together with simulation models that allows recreating different variations of colorblindness, allowing people with a trichromat vision, to be able to perceive the environment in the same way as a person with colorblindness does (Hans Brettel, 1997).

The use of these simulation models has recently been extended to applications in smart phones by using the cellphone camera taking real time photographs an casting them to the device screen, allowing to experiment colorblindness, such as the Chromatic Vision SimulatorTM (CVS) application, developed by Kazunori Asada in 2012. This application cites the model in (Hans Brettel, 1997) y (Tomoyuki Ohkubo, 2010).

The simulations in Figure 1 shows how the color spectrum is perceived by people with normal vision and the different variants of dichromacy simulated with the CVS application.

Occurrence Rate of Color Blindness

Color blindness due to congenital causes associated with genetic inheritance occurs in about 10% of the population. The severity of this condition is lower for most of

Figure 1. Perception of the color spectrum with variants of colorblindness obtained with CVS
Source: own/authors

cases of colorblindness and the most critical variants of this disability have lower occurrence; Table 1 shows the worldwide prevalence of the different variants of colorblindness (Colblindor, 2016; Chieko Kato, 2013).

There are several tests for colorblindness detection, some of them require medical analysis, as well as specialized equipment, but providing high accuracy compared with the other tests, other tests do not require prior medical preparation and the results may ensure the detection of colorblindness, but medical diagnosis is recommended for concluding results (Richmond Products, 2016; Colblindor, 2016; Toke Bek, 2000).

Tests for colorblindness are divided into four diagnostic areas: anomaloscopy, placement tests, pseudochromatic plates, and electronic tests (Colblindor, 2016).

Ishihara plates are the most common pseudochromatic plates and its popularity made them an icon for this disability (Colblindor, 2016). Ishihara test is made by presenting to the patient several plates with colors that people with colorblindness confuse, so they are based on the theory of co-punctual points, the plates are discs with numbers that are confused with the background, mistaken identified plates are taken as a reference to determine the variant of colorblindness. Ishihara plates are designed for the detection of protanopia, protanomaly, deuteranopia and deuteranomaly. Figure 2 shows 42 Ishihara plate (Ishihara, 1972).

Main problems of colorblind people are related to identify and perceive colors in a confuse region. There are several efforts using digital technologies to assist colorblind people with those problems and augmented reality (the process of acquiring images modify them for retransmitting in order to mix virtual elements with the real world, which include marking the confuse region for colorblind people) have allowed help people with disabilities (Enrico Tanuwidjaja, 2014; Young-geun Kim, 2014).

Table 1. Occurrence rate of Color blindness

Colorblindness quantity of cones variant	Color cone sub variant	Occurrence M/F	
Monochromacy	Achromatopsia	0.00003%	
Dichromacy	Deuteranopia	1.27%	0.01%
	Protanopia	1.01%	0.02%
	Tritanopia	0.0001%	
Anomalous Trichromacy	Deuteranomaly	4.63%	0.36%
	Protanomaly	1.08%	0.03%
	Tritanomaly	0.0002%	

Source: Colorblindor, 2016

Figure 2. Ishihara 42 plate taking from
Source: Ishihara, 1972

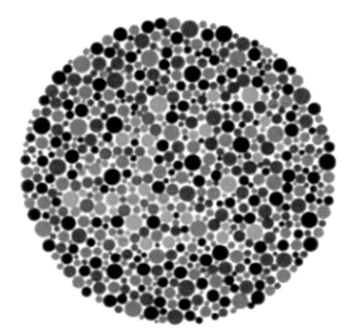

An alternative used for assisting colorblind people whit colors that they cannot distinguish well. Is to use a common device as an android cellphone for real time acquisition images and recoloring of them in pixels detected as confuse colors, then images are retransmitted to colorblind people so that confuse regions of colors be identified.

Confusion colors detection require a processing algorithm This is a research field where artificial intelligence have shown good results on classification and detection of parameters (Engelbrecht, 2007). Artificial Neural Networks (ANNs) are an Artificial Intelligence technique inspired on mathematical models for understanding the biological nervous system ANNs can perform complex tasks through learning that can be either supervised when input data is labeled or unsupervised when it is not (Engelbrecht, 2007).

Objective

In this paper is proposed the development of an application for assisting colorblind people using a cellphone camera for acquiring images that are send to a computer and then for being processed to identify the regions of color labeled as confuse colors, the classification stage is done with ANNs that are trained using a supervised algorithm called gradient descent backpropagation an Ishihara plates are used as training input data for select colors that are labeled as confused for colorblind people.

BACKGROUND

Assisting people with disabilities by using augmented reality is a research field of interest and several works are beginning to contribute in this area, such as those shown in Table 2.

Since colorblind people cannot perceive confused colors, a digital camera performs image acquisition of the surroundings for identification of confusing colors. The digital camera captures the energy from the light, just as the eyes do with the cones and rods, by using sensory units that react to the basic colors (Figure 3), Red, Green and Blue (known as the RGB color spectrum) and produce signals that can be transformed into digital data (Gonzalez & Woods, 2001; Martín Montes Rivera, 2016).

Pixels indicate the size of an image and its quality, but color representation subdivides each pixel into three numerical parameters with n bits of resolution depending from the analog to digital converter ADC. These values can be represented in a three-dimensional space, with its RGB representation as shown in Figure 4 (Martín Montes Rivera, 2016).

There are other color representations for color classification in color digital images as Hue, Saturation and Value (HSV), Hue, Saturation and Intensity (HSI), Hue, Saturation Mixture (HSM), CIELab (L is the lightness and parameter and a for green to red parameter and b for blue to yellow parameter), among others. All of this transformations have specific applications for example HSV which is mainly

Table 2. Related works to colorblindness using augmented reality

Title	Year
Chroma: A Wearable Augmented-Reality Solution for Color-Blindness	2015
A Real-time Color-matching Method Based on Smartphones For Color-blind people	2014
Implementation of assistance system for people with colorblindness	2013
Implementing Speech Feature for Embedded System to Support Color Blind People	2011
Development of a Color-assisted Vision System for Persons with Colorvision Deficiency	2010

Source: own/authors

Figure 3. RGB perceiving unit taking from
Source: Gonzalez & Woods, 2001

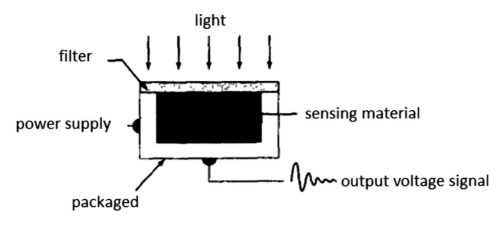

Figure 4. RGB spectrum with 8 bits taking from
Source: Martín Montes Rivera, 2016

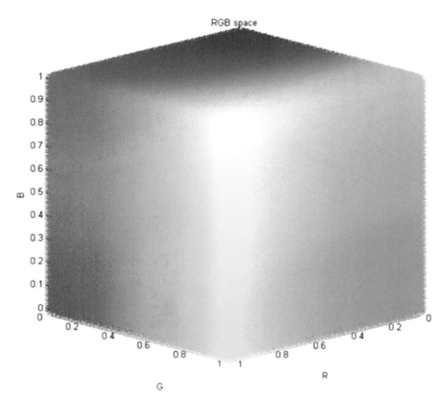

used for color classification, nevertheless, every color transformation require several iterations for changing every pixel of an image to its new representation, since RGB space is directly obtained from cameras require less computational power for color classification, but the complexity for performing the classification is increased, because this space require no linear operations for classification, although ANNs deals well with this kind of tasks (Martín Montes Rivera, 2016).

ANNs are mathematical models for neural networks in the nervous system. Real neurons have inputs called dendrites and its output is called axon which either could be activated or disactivated depending from the dendrites and the soma is the body of the cell that classify those inputs. Synapse is the number of dendrites linked to a specific path, this number is increased for maximizing communication between commonly used links. ANNs first architecture proposed by McCuloch and Pits in 1943 has inputs x_i and output y and synapse is reproduced with w_i weights, as shown in Figure 5. The activation function for McCuloch and Pits neuron is shown in equation (1) (Nguyen, Prasad, Walker, & Walker, 2003).

$$F\left(z\right) = \begin{cases} 1 & z \geq \theta \\ 0 & z < \theta \end{cases} \tag{1}$$

where z is the total input to the neuron with its prior w_i weights, as in equation (2).

$$z = \sum_{i=1}^{n} x_i w_i \tag{2}$$

Figure 5. Comparative between McCuloch and Pits ANNs and biological neural network
Source: own/authors

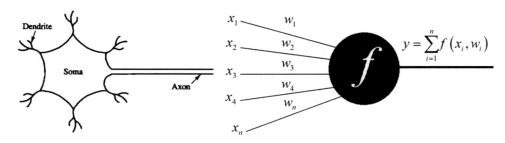

Despite of McCuloch and Pits neuron was the first introduced, several new ANNs architectures and models were developed, Hebb and perceptron neurons were the first ANNs with supervised training algorithms but they also were highly limited because they could not train hidden layers required in more complex tasks (Nguyen, Prasad, Walker, & Walker, 2003).

Backpropagation Gradient Descent is a very popular learning rule that allows to train ANNs with hidden layers, the ANNs with backpropagation initially used a sigmoid activation function with y outputs in range $0 \leq y \leq 1$, differing from perceptron and Hebb neurons that has only binary outputs, nevertheless, there have appeared other activation functions with their own proprieties (Nguyen, Prasad, Walker, & Walker, 2003; Uday Pratap Singh, 2018). In this paper is used a hyperbolic sigmoid activation function (3) combined with a linear activation function (4), because together are a good function approximator for every function with finite discontinuities (Valeriy Dubrovin, 2000; Demuth & Beale, 1998).

$$\tan sh(wpb_{ijk}) = \frac{2}{\left(1 + e^{-2wpb_{ijk}}\right) - 1} \tag{3}$$

$$linear(wpb_{ij}) = wpb_{ij} \tag{4}$$

Once that previous ANNs is constructed then is trained using Backpropagation algorithm learning rule which can be explained by considering architecture in Figure 6. Updates of weights with are performed with equations (5) and (6).

Figure 6. Architecture for Backpropagation formulation
Source: own/authors

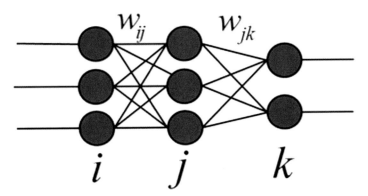

$$w_{ij} = w_{ij} + \alpha x_i \delta_j \tag{5}$$

$$w_{jk} = w_{jk} + \alpha y_j \delta_k \tag{6}$$

With $\delta_k = \dfrac{\partial y_k}{\partial x_k} e_k$ and $\delta_j = \dfrac{\partial y_j}{\partial x_j} \sum_{k=1}^{n} w_{jk} \delta_k$ with $e_k = d_k - y_k$ where d_k is the desired output in the y_k output.

Support and Similar Works

The main support for using ANNs in this first study is based on the results obtained for color classification tasks using artificial neural networks algorithms, which efficiency reach 99.8%, while other techniques have lower efficiency results as described in (Saeed, Ahmad, Alsadi, Ross, & Rizvi, 2014).

Other alternatives for classifying colors obtain efficiency levels under 92% efficiency like described in (Nasiri, Yazdi, Moulavi, Rouhani, & Shargh, 2008)

Works that use this processing techniques applied to assisting colorblind people include: The work in (Fuller & Sadovnik, 2017), where confuse colors are identified and isolated from the image but the results do not mix reality with labels or marks for the identified pixels resulting in images that are not natural for the user. Other work that uses processing images techniques is the described in (Enrico Tanuwidjaja, 2014), marking pixels only whit white color and retransmitting those pixels to the user allowing them to pass Ishihara plates but with images of lower quality and with no natural perception because of the change of color in pixels.

METHODOLOGY

The first part for implementing the proposed algorithm is to generate the labeled training data, this is made by a person with trichromat vision, that edit several Ishihara plates, marking the numbers of the plates or the background depending from the variant of colorblindness and the plate color. Colors marked for deuteranopia are green and brown, and red and orange are identified for protanopia. The images are marked by changing to white all pixels identified as confused colors and any other color remains equal, however user can mark colors in black in they are no confusing colors for help him to distinguish very close colors.

The proposed architecture for ANNs has a function $\tan sh(\mathrm{x})$ for its input and hidden layer and a $linear(\mathrm{x})$ function for its output layer. First input of the layer given with equation (7), where k represents the weight of neuron j in the layer i and bias b always get $k = 1$, since there is only a bias per layer.

$$wpb_{1j} = R \times w_{1j1} + G \times w_{1j2} + Bw_{1j3} + b_{1j1} \tag{7}$$

Second and third layer has input parameter given by equation (8)

$$wpb_{ijk} = A_{(i-1)1} \times w_{ij1} + A_{(i-1)2}w_{ij2} \times + A_{(i-1)3} \times w_{ij3} + b_{ij1} \tag{8}$$

where A_{ij} is the neuron j output in the layer i and for first and second $A_{ij} = \tan sh(wpb_{ij})$ in equation (3), and for the last layer $A_{ij} = linear(wpb_{ij})$ in equation (4) .

After that neural network architecture is ready is trained using gradient descent backpropagation rule, as described in background section, then all the resulting pixels detected as confusing colors are increased in their bright but considering a τ threshold ANNs output is in range $(0,1)$, threshold is used with ANNs output according to equation (9).

$$A_{31} > \tau \tag{9}$$

Pixels are changed in bright according to equation (10), allowing to modify parameters κ, λ and o for a correct perception of colorblind people without get a disturbing image, allowing to get more natural images for the user by modifying only the bright of the pixels and retaining proprieties of images as colors and shadows that colorblind people usually see.

$$\begin{bmatrix} NR \\ NG \\ NB \end{bmatrix} = \begin{bmatrix} \kappa \times R \\ \lambda \times G \\ o \times B \end{bmatrix} \tag{10}$$

RESULTS

The input data labeled is shown in Figure 7. This several pictures are divided in two classes those that are direct inputs used in the neurons which does not have any alteration and those interpreted as desired outputs having modifications in their pixels changing them to white when the ANNs output must be activated, and remaining on its color or changing to black if the ANNs output must remain inhibit.

Training of neural network was performed according to algorithm described in background section using MATLAB™ since it has implemented the required algorithm and architecture obtained with this software is shown in Figure 8.

The training results for green, brown, red and orange colors are shown in Figure 9 with minimal errors evaluated with Mean Square Error (MSE) as training function.

Figure 7. Labeled input data for training
Source: own/authors

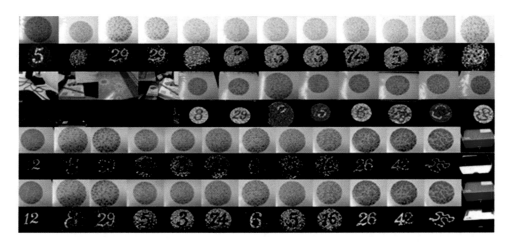

Figure 8. ANN architecture implemented in MATLABTM
Source: own/authors

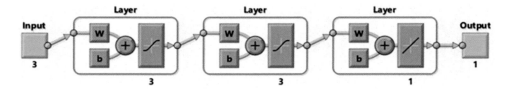

Figure 9. ANN training results per color. Source: own/authors

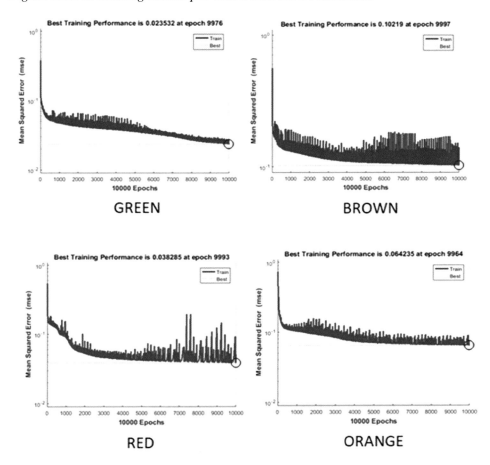

Processed images after identifying marked colors with $\kappa = 1.7, \lambda = 1.7, o = 0.25$ for equation (10), produce images with increase in bright for confusing colors. The test in the image in Figure 10 shows the results compared with a colorblind simulation algorithm for understand how a colorblind person perceives the proposed algorithm.

The table 3 shows a comparative between the obtained results with and without use the proposed algorithm for assistance during the Ishihara test, were LP means that is seen a line path and N means that is nothing seen.

Figure 10. Output results after processing algorithm
Source: own/authors

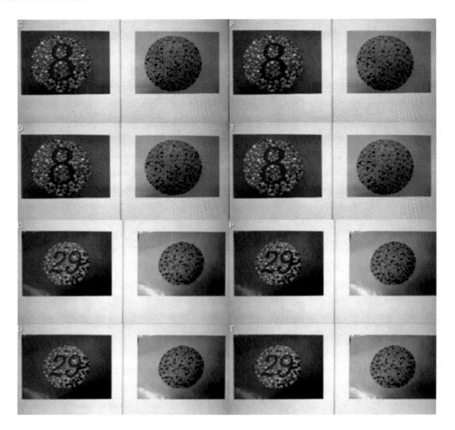

CONCLUSION

The proposed algorithm classifies colors using ANNs with Ishihara plates as input data for teach an intelligent system to identify the colors in confuse regions for colorblind people, the train is reached with a minimal training error described with MSE, validation checks are performed during the training stage for verify a successful training.

Processed images achieve its expected result since a colorblind patient can fully identify the plates in the Ishihara Test in real time by using its cellphone as acquiring images device.

Table 3. Comparative of results in Ishihara plates by patient with and without proposed algorithm

Plate number	Correct plate	Plate seen without algorithm				Plate seen with algorithm			
		P1	P2	P3	P4	P1	P2	P3	P4
1	12	12	12	12	12	12	12	12	12
2	8	3	N	3	N	8	8	8	8
3	29	29	N	N	N	29	29	29	29
4	5	N	N	N	N	5	5	5	5
5	3	N	8	N	N	3	3	3	3
6	15	N	15	15	N	15	15	15	15
7	74	N	21	84	N	74	74	74	74
8	6	N	N	N	N	6	6	6	6
9	45	N	N	N	N	45	45	45	45
10	5	N	8	11	N	5	5	5	5
11	7	N	7	7	N	7	7	7	7
12	16	N	N	16	N	16	16	16	16
13	73	N	N	N	N	73	73	73	73
14	LP	N	N	N	LP	LP	LP	LP	LP
15	LP	N	N	N	LP	LP	LP	LP	LP
16	26	N	26	26	2	26	26	26	26
17	42	N	42	42	4	42	42	42	42
18	LP	N	LP	LP	LP	LP	LP	LP	LP
19	LP	N	N	N	LP	LP	LP	LP	LP
20	LP	N	N	N	N	LP	LP	LP	LP
21	LP	N	N	N	N	LP	LP	LP	LP
22	LP	N	N	N	N	LP	LP	LP	LP
23	LP	N	N	N	N	LP	LP	LP	LP
24	LP	LP	LP	N	LP	LP	LP	LP	LP

Source: own/authors

The images processed can be perceived correctly by a person with colorblindness as by a person with normal view, with they own common vision, allowing them to identify confuse regions with colors that are difficult to distinguish for colorblind people.

Perception of images with the proposed technique retransmit pictures retaining color and shadows while increasing bright so that the processed images be comfortable for the user.

FUTURE WORK

For concluding results future work will compare several cases of colorblind people using the proposed algorithm in order to guarantee good results when colorblindness is diagnosed.

Several other machine learning algorithms could be tested for find which obtain better results when detecting confusing colors for colorblind people.

ACKNOWLEDGMENT

To Francisco Montes Betancourt, Adrian Pelayo García, Sergio Camarillo Barba and David Gómez Almaraz colorblind patients that has tested the proposed algorithm and help to improve it with its recommendations for perceive correctly the Ishihara plates.

REFERENCES

Antonio Tagarelli, A. P. (2004). Colour blindness in everyday life and car driving. *Acta Ophthalmologica Scandinavica*, 82(4), 436–442. doi:10.1111/j.1395-3907.2004.00283.x PMID:15291938

Chieko Kato, K.-s. (2013). Comprehending Color Images for Color Barrier-Free via Factor Analysis Technique. *International Conference on Software Engineering, Artificial Intelligence, Networking and Parallel/Distributed Computing*, 478-483.

Colblindor. (2016). Obtenido de http://www.color-blindness.com/wp-content/documents/Color-Blind-Essentials.pdf

Deeb, S. S. (2004). Molecular genetics of colour vision deficiencies. *Clinical & Experimental Optometry*, 87(4-5), 224–229. doi:10.1111/j.1444-0938.2004.tb05052.x PMID:15312026

Demuth, H., & Beale, M. (1998). *Neural Network Toolbox for Use with MATLAB*. MathWorks Inc.

Engelbrecht, A. P. (2007). *Computacional Intelligence. Sudafrica*. Wiley. doi:10.1002/9780470512517

Enrico Tanuwidjaja, D. H. (2014). Chroma: A Wearable Augmented-Reality Solution for Color Blindness. In *Proceedings of the 2014 ACM International Joint Conference on Pervasive and Ubiquitous Computing* (pp. 799-810). Google. 10.1145/2632048.2632091

Fuller, T., & Sadovnik, A. (2017). Image level color classification for colorblind assistance. In *International Conference on Image Processing (ICIP).* (pp. 1985-1989). IEEE. 10.1109/ICIP.2017.8296629

Gonzalez, R. C., & Woods, R. E. (2001). *Digital Image Processing.* Prentice Hall.

Hans Brettel, F. V. (1997). Computerized simulation of color appearance for dichromats. *Journal of the Optical Society of America*, *14*(10), 2647–2655. doi:10.1364/JOSAA.14.002647 PMID:9316278

Hatem, M., & Marey, N. A. (2015). Ishihara Electronic Color Blindness Test: An Evaluation Study. *Ophthalmology Research: An International Journal*, 67-75.

Ishihara, S. (1972). *Test for colour-blindness.* Tokyo: Kanehara Shuppan Co. Ltd.

Kim, Y., & Kim, W. (2014). Implementation of Augmented Reality System for Smartphone Advertisements. *International Journal of Multimedia and Ubiquitous Engineering*, *9*(2), 385–392. doi:10.14257/ijmue.2014.9.2.39

Martín Montes Rivera, A. P. (2016). Comparative between RGB and HSV color representations for color segmentation when it is applied with artificial neural networks and evolutionary algorithms. In A. R. Ma. de Lourdes Sánchez Guerrero (Ed.), Avances en las Tecnologías de la Información (pp. 611-629). Ciudad de México, México: Alfa-Omega.

Nasiri, J., Yazdi, H., Moulavi, M., Rouhani, M., & Shargh, A. (2008). *A PSO tuning approach for lip detection on color images.* Computer Modelling and Simulation IEEE. doi:10.1109/EMS.2008.98

Nguyen, H. T., Prasad, N. R., Walker, C. L., & Walker, E. A. (2003). *A First Course in Fuzzy and Neural Control.* Chapman and Hall.

Porrero, J. G., & J. H. (2005). *Anatomía Humana.* Madrid: McGraw-Hill Interamericana.

Richmond Products. (2016). *Richmond Products.* Obtenido de Color Vision Deficiency A Concise Tutorial for Optometry and Ophthalmology: http://www.richmondproducts. com/files/8013/0590/4424/Color_Vision_Deficiency_Tutorial_042511.pdf

Robson, D. (2016). *BBC.* Obtenido de Mundo: http://www.bbc.com/mundo/ noticias/2014/09/140911_vert_fut_mujeres_vision_superhumana_finde_dv

Ruki Harwahyu, R. F. (2011). Implementing Speech Feature for Embedded System to Support Color Blind People. *First International Conference on Informatics and Computational Intelligence.* 10.1109/ICI.2011.49

Saeed, U., Ahmad, S., Alsadi, J., Ross, D., & Rizvi, G. (2014). Implementation of neural network for color properties of polycarbonates. In AIP Conference Proceedings (vol. 1593, pp. 56–59). American Institute of Physics. doi:10.1063/1.4873733

Tanaka, K. D. (2015). A colour to birds and to humans: Why is it so different? *J Ornithol*, S434–S440.

Toke Bek, M. K. (2000). Quantitative anomaloscopy and optical coherence tomography scanning in central serous chorioretinopathy. *Acta Ophthalmologica Scandinavica*, 632–637. PMID:11167221

Tomoyuki Ohkubo, K. K. (2010). Development of a Time-sharing-based Color-assisted Vision System for Persons with Color-vision Deficiency. *SICE Annual Conference*, 2499-2503.

Uday Pratap Singh, S. J. (2018). Optimization of neural network for nonlinear discrete time system using modified quaternion firefly algorithm: Case study of Indian currency exchange rate prediction. *Soft Computing*, 8(8), 2667–2681. doi:10.100700500-017-2522-x

Valeriy Dubrovin, S. S. (2000). Neural Network Method in Plant Spectral Recognition. In R. S. Muttiah (Ed.), From Laboratory Spectroscopy to Remotely Sensed Spectra of Terrestrial of Terrestrial Ecosystems (pp. 147-159). Kluwer Academic Publishers.

Related Readings

To continue IGI Global's long-standing tradition of advancing innovation through emerging research, please find below a compiled list of recommended IGI Global book chapters and journal articles in the areas of blind and visually impaired, teaching aids, and assistive technologies. These related readings will provide additional information and guidance to further enrich your knowledge and assist you with your own research.

Afyf, A., Bellarbi, L., Latrach, M., Gaviot, E., Camberlein, L., Sennouni, M. A., & Yaakoui, N. (2018). Wearable Antennas: Breast Cancer Detection. In S. Delabrida Silva, R. Rabelo Oliveira, & A. Loureiro (Eds.), *Examining Developments and Applications of Wearable Devices in Modern Society* (pp. 161–202). Hershey, PA: IGI Global. doi:10.4018/978-1-5225-3290-3.ch007

Amhag, L. (2016). Mobile Technologies for Student Centered Learning in a Distance Higher Education Program. In J. Holland (Ed.), *Wearable Technology and Mobile Innovations for Next-Generation Education* (pp. 184–199). Hershey, PA: IGI Global. doi:10.4018/978-1-5225-0069-8.ch010

Amorim, V. J., Delabrida Silva, S. E., & Oliveira, R. A. (2018). Wearables Operating Systems: A Comparison Based on Relevant Constraints. In S. Delabrida Silva, R. Rabelo Oliveira, & A. Loureiro (Eds.), *Examining Developments and Applications of Wearable Devices in Modern Society* (pp. 86–106). Hershey, PA: IGI Global. doi:10.4018/978-1-5225-3290-3.ch004

Anderson, C. L., & Anderson, K. M. (2019). Practical Examples of Using Switch-Adapted and Battery-Powered Technology to Benefit Persons With Disabilities. In S. Ikuta (Ed.), *Handmade Teaching Materials for Students With Disabilities* (pp. 212–230). Hershey, PA: IGI Global. doi:10.4018/978-1-5225-6240-5.ch009

Angelova, R. A. (2018). Wearable Technologies for Helping Human Thermophysiological Comfort. In S. Delabrida Silva, R. Rabelo Oliveira, & A. Loureiro (Eds.), *Examining Developments and Applications of Wearable Devices in Modern Society* (pp. 203–231). Hershey, PA: IGI Global. doi:10.4018/978-1-5225-3290-3.ch008

Arpaci, I. (2016). Design and Development of Educational Multimedia: The Software Development Process for Mobile Learning. In J. Holland (Ed.), *Wearable Technology and Mobile Innovations for Next-Generation Education* (pp. 147–165). Hershey, PA: IGI Global. doi:10.4018/978-1-5225-0069-8.ch008

Baker, A., Asino, T., Xiu, Y., & Fulgencio, J. L. (2017). Logistical Issues With OER Initiative in a K-12 Environment. In M. Mills & D. Wake (Eds.), *Empowering Learners With Mobile Open-Access Learning Initiatives* (pp. 98–119). Hershey, PA: IGI Global. doi:10.4018/978-1-5225-2122-8.ch007

Barker, B. S., Nugent, G., Grandgenett, N., Keshwani, J., Nelson, C. A., & Leduc-Mills, B. (2016). Developing an Elementary Engineering Education Program through Problem-Based Wearable Technologies Activities. In J. Holland (Ed.), *Wearable Technology and Mobile Innovations for Next-Generation Education* (pp. 269–294). Hershey, PA: IGI Global. doi:10.4018/978-1-5225-0069-8.ch014

Bello-Bravo, J., Lutomia, A. N., Abbott, E., Mazur, R., Mocumbe, S., & Pittendrigh, B. R. (2017). Making Agricultural Learning Accessible: Examining Gender in the Use of Animations via Mobile Phones. In M. Mills & D. Wake (Eds.), *Empowering Learners With Mobile Open-Access Learning Initiatives* (pp. 47–73). Hershey, PA: IGI Global. doi:10.4018/978-1-5225-2122-8.ch005

Blau, I. (2019). Real-Time Mobile Assessment of Learning: Insights From an Experiment With Middle School Students From Remedial, Midstream, and Excellence Tracks. In A. Forkosh Baruch & H. Meishar Tal (Eds.), *Mobile Technologies in Educational Organizations* (pp. 283–301). Hershey, PA: IGI Global. doi:10.4018/978-1-5225-8106-2.ch014

Blonder, R., & Waldman, R. (2019). The Role of a WhatsApp Group of a Professional Learning Community of Chemistry Teachers in the Development of Their Knowledge. In A. Forkosh Baruch & H. Meishar Tal (Eds.), *Mobile Technologies in Educational Organizations* (pp. 117–140). Hershey, PA: IGI Global. doi:10.4018/978-1-5225-8106-2.ch007

Butler, M. S., & Luebbers, P. E. (2016). Health and Fitness Wearables. In J. Holland (Ed.), *Wearable Technology and Mobile Innovations for Next-Generation Education* (pp. 58–78). Hershey, PA: IGI Global. doi:10.4018/978-1-5225-0069-8.ch004

Related Readings

Chamblin, M. (2018). Thinking It Through: Using the ADAPT Strategy to Differentiate and Adapt Instruction. In P. Epler (Ed.), *Instructional Strategies in General Education and Putting the Individuals With Disabilities Act (IDEA) Into Practice* (pp. 167–195). Hershey, PA: IGI Global. doi:10.4018/978-1-5225-3111-1.ch006

Chappel, J. (2017). "With Tension Comes a Little Work": Motivation and Safety in Online Peer Review. In M. Mills & D. Wake (Eds.), *Empowering Learners With Mobile Open-Access Learning Initiatives* (pp. 238–261). Hershey, PA: IGI Global. doi:10.4018/978-1-5225-2122-8.ch013

Chen, Y., & Zhang, Y. (2019). Culture and Context Impact on Mobile Tech Application in Organizational Learning: Case Study of UK Higher Education Institution and Chinese State-Owned Enterprise. In A. Forkosh Baruch & H. Meishar Tal (Eds.), *Mobile Technologies in Educational Organizations* (pp. 142–169). Hershey, PA: IGI Global. doi:10.4018/978-1-5225-8106-2.ch008

Choudhury, A., & Sarma, K. K. (2019). Visual Gesture-Based Character Recognition Systems for Design of Assistive Technologies for People With Special Necessities. In S. Ikuta (Ed.), *Handmade Teaching Materials for Students With Disabilities* (pp. 294–315). Hershey, PA: IGI Global. doi:10.4018/978-1-5225-6240-5.ch013

Coffman, T. L., & Klinger, M. B. (2019). Mobile Technologies for Making Meaning in Education: Using Augmented Reality to Connect Learning. In A. Forkosh Baruch & H. Meishar Tal (Eds.), *Mobile Technologies in Educational Organizations* (pp. 64–84). Hershey, PA: IGI Global. doi:10.4018/978-1-5225-8106-2.ch004

Cohen, A., & Ezra, O. (2019). Contextualized MALL in Target and Non-Target Countries: Mobile Activity Evaluation. In A. Forkosh Baruch & H. Meishar Tal (Eds.), *Mobile Technologies in Educational Organizations* (pp. 170–191). Hershey, PA: IGI Global. doi:10.4018/978-1-5225-8106-2.ch009

D'Angelo, T., Delabrida Silva, S. E., Oliveira, R. A., & Loureiro, A. A. (2018). Development of a Low-Cost Augmented Reality Head-Mounted Display Prototype. In S. Delabrida Silva, R. Rabelo Oliveira, & A. Loureiro (Eds.), *Examining Developments and Applications of Wearable Devices in Modern Society* (pp. 1–28). Hershey, PA: IGI Global. doi:10.4018/978-1-5225-3290-3.ch001

Dalton, E. M. (2019). Diversity, Disability, and Addressing the Varied Needs of Learners: Guiding Material Design and Instruction. In S. Ikuta (Ed.), *Handmade Teaching Materials for Students With Disabilities* (pp. 1–19). Hershey, PA: IGI Global. doi:10.4018/978-1-5225-6240-5.ch001

Dias, J. R., Penha, R., Morgado, L., Alves da Veiga, P., Carvalho, E. S., & Fernandes-Marcos, A. (2019). Tele-Media-Art:Feasibility Tests of Web-Based Dance Education for the Blind Using Kinect and Sound Synthesis of Motion. *International Journal of Technology and Human Interaction*, *15*(2), 11–28. doi:10.4018/IJTHI.2019040102

Doi, K., & Nishimura, T. (2019). Production Method of Readable Tactile Map With Vocal Guidance Function for the Visually Impaired. In S. Ikuta (Ed.), *Handmade Teaching Materials for Students With Disabilities* (pp. 316–337). Hershey, PA: IGI Global. doi:10.4018/978-1-5225-6240-5.ch014

Drivet, A. (2016). Wearable Cameras. In J. Holland (Ed.), *Wearable Technology and Mobile Innovations for Next-Generation Education* (pp. 95–121). Hershey, PA: IGI Global. doi:10.4018/978-1-5225-0069-8.ch006

Epler, P. L. (2018). Teaching Students With Specific Learning Disabilities in the General Education Classroom. In P. Epler (Ed.), *Instructional Strategies in General Education and Putting the Individuals With Disabilities Act (IDEA) Into Practice* (pp. 39–74). Hershey, PA: IGI Global. doi:10.4018/978-1-5225-3111-1.ch002

Epler, P. L. (2018). Working With Attention-Deficit Disorder, Attention-Deficit/Hyperactivity Disorder, and Twice-Exceptional Students. In P. Epler (Ed.), *Instructional Strategies in General Education and Putting the Individuals With Disabilities Act (IDEA) Into Practice* (pp. 75–92). Hershey, PA: IGI Global. doi:10.4018/978-1-5225-3111-1.ch003

Epler, P. L. (2019). Strategies for Teaching Math to Middle and High School Students With Special Needs. In S. Ikuta (Ed.), *Handmade Teaching Materials for Students With Disabilities* (pp. 232–252). Hershey, PA: IGI Global. doi:10.4018/978-1-5225-6240-5.ch010

Ferguson, B. T. (2019). Supporting Affective Development of Children With Disabilities Through Moral Dilemmas. In S. Ikuta (Ed.), *Handmade Teaching Materials for Students With Disabilities* (pp. 253–275). Hershey, PA: IGI Global. doi:10.4018/978-1-5225-6240-5.ch011

Fishelson, R. I. (2019). Time for a Change: Designing a Mobile Application to Assist People With Intellectual Disabilities. In A. Forkosh Baruch & H. Meishar Tal (Eds.), *Mobile Technologies in Educational Organizations* (pp. 211–232). Hershey, PA: IGI Global. doi:10.4018/978-1-5225-8106-2.ch011

Related Readings

Gallavan, N. P., Huffman, S., & Shaw, E. C. (2017). Ensuring Ethics and Equity With Classroom Assessments and Mobile Technology: Advancing Online Education. In M. Mills & D. Wake (Eds.), *Empowering Learners With Mobile Open-Access Learning Initiatives* (pp. 193–214). Hershey, PA: IGI Global. doi:10.4018/978-1-5225-2122-8.ch011

Gallup, J., Kocaoz, O. E., & Serianni, B. (2019). Virtual Mediums Used as a Conduit for Soft-Skill Development: A Naturalistic and Innovative Approach – Virtual Mediums to Support Soft-Skills. In S. Ikuta (Ed.), *Handmade Teaching Materials for Students With Disabilities* (pp. 276–292). Hershey, PA: IGI Global. doi:10.4018/978-1-5225-6240-5.ch012

Gallup, J. L., Ray, B. B., & Bennett, C. A. (2019). Leveraging Mobile Technologies to Support Active Learning for All Students: Smartphones to Support Learning. In A. Forkosh Baruch & H. Meishar Tal (Eds.), *Mobile Technologies in Educational Organizations* (pp. 302–326). Hershey, PA: IGI Global. doi:10.4018/978-1-5225-8106-2.ch015

Gibson, R. (2016). Wearable Technologies in Academic Information Search. In J. Holland (Ed.), *Wearable Technology and Mobile Innovations for Next-Generation Education* (pp. 122–146). Hershey, PA: IGI Global. doi:10.4018/978-1-5225-0069-8.ch007

Grant, M. C. (2018). IDEA and Inclusive Education: Issues, Implications, and Practices. In P. Epler (Ed.), *Instructional Strategies in General Education and Putting the Individuals With Disabilities Act (IDEA) Into Practice* (pp. 1–38). Hershey, PA: IGI Global. doi:10.4018/978-1-5225-3111-1.ch001

Hariharan, R. (2018). Wearable Internet of Things. In S. Delabrida Silva, R. Rabelo Oliveira, & A. Loureiro (Eds.), *Examining Developments and Applications of Wearable Devices in Modern Society* (pp. 29–57). Hershey, PA: IGI Global. doi:10.4018/978-1-5225-3290-3.ch002

Hassan, A., & Privitera, D. S. (2016). Google AdSense as a Mobile Technology in Education. In J. Holland (Ed.), *Wearable Technology and Mobile Innovations for Next-Generation Education* (pp. 200–223). Hershey, PA: IGI Global. doi:10.4018/978-1-5225-0069-8.ch011

Herring, J. (2017). Empowering High-Needs Students With Problem-Based Learning Through Mobile Technology. In M. Mills & D. Wake (Eds.), *Empowering Learners With Mobile Open-Access Learning Initiatives* (pp. 1–12). Hershey, PA: IGI Global. doi:10.4018/978-1-5225-2122-8.ch001

HingTing, K. L., & Di Loreto, I. (2017). A Participatory Design Approach with Visually Impaired People for the Design of an Art Exhibition. *International Journal of Sociotechnology and Knowledge Development*, 9(4), 43–57. doi:10.4018/IJSKD.2017100104

Hopcan, S., Tokel, S. T., Karasu, N., & Aykut, Ç. (2019). Design and Development of a Mobile Writing Application for Students With Dysgraphia. In A. Forkosh Baruch & H. Meishar Tal (Eds.), *Mobile Technologies in Educational Organizations* (pp. 233–262). Hershey, PA: IGI Global. doi:10.4018/978-1-5225-8106-2.ch012

Hossain, G. (2017). Design Analytics of Complex Communication Systems Involving Two Different Sensory Disabilities. *International Journal of Healthcare Information Systems and Informatics*, 12(2), 65–80. doi:10.4018/IJHISI.2017040104

Hudgins, T., & Holland, J. L. (2016). Digital Badges: Tracking Knowledge Acquisition within an Innovation Framework. In J. Holland (Ed.), *Wearable Technology and Mobile Innovations for Next-Generation Education* (pp. 80–94). Hershey, PA: IGI Global. doi:10.4018/978-1-5225-0069-8.ch005

Iaquinta, R., & Iaquinta, T. (2016). Education Technology Disposable Information. In J. Holland (Ed.), *Wearable Technology and Mobile Innovations for Next-Generation Education* (pp. 20–36). Hershey, PA: IGI Global. doi:10.4018/978-1-5225-0069-8.ch002

Ikuta, S., Nagano, S., Sato, E. T., Kasai, M., Ezoe, T., Mori, K., & Kaneko, C. (2019). Original Teaching Materials and School Activities With E-Books Containing Media Overlays. In S. Ikuta (Ed.), *Handmade Teaching Materials for Students With Disabilities* (pp. 76–110). Hershey, PA: IGI Global. doi:10.4018/978-1-5225-6240-5.ch004

Ikuta, S., Yamashita, S., Higo, H., Tomiyama, J., Saotome, N., Sudo, S., ... Watanuki, M. (2019). Original Teaching Materials and School Activities With Multimedia-Enabled Dot Codes. In S. Ikuta (Ed.), *Handmade Teaching Materials for Students With Disabilities* (pp. 50–75). Hershey, PA: IGI Global. doi:10.4018/978-1-5225-6240-5.ch003

Ishitobi, R., Nemoto, F., Sugita, Y., Nakamura, S., Iijima, T., Takatsu, A., ... Ikuta, S. (2019). Original Teaching Materials and School Activities for Students With an Intellectual Disability. In S. Ikuta (Ed.), *Handmade Teaching Materials for Students With Disabilities* (pp. 111–131). Hershey, PA: IGI Global. doi:10.4018/978-1-5225-6240-5.ch005

Jackson, N. H. (2017). Fusing Culturally Responsive Teaching, Place Conscious Education, and Problem-Based Learning With Mobile Technologies: Sparking Change. In M. Mills & D. Wake (Eds.), *Empowering Learners With Mobile Open-Access Learning Initiatives* (pp. 288–306). Hershey, PA: IGI Global. doi:10.4018/978-1-5225-2122-8.ch015

Juliana, I., Izuagbe, R., Itsekor, V., Fagbohun, M. O., Asaolu, A., & Nwokeoma, M. N. (2018). The Role of the School Library in Empowering Visually Impaired Children With Lifelong Information Literacy Skills. In P. Epler (Ed.), *Instructional Strategies in General Education and Putting the Individuals With Disabilities Act (IDEA) Into Practice* (pp. 245–271). Hershey, PA: IGI Global. doi:10.4018/978-1-5225-3111-1.ch009

Khalifa, S., Lan, G., Hassan, M., Hu, W., & Seneviratne, A. (2018). Human Context Detection From Kinetic Energy Harvesting Wearables. In S. Delabrida Silva, R. Rabelo Oliveira, & A. Loureiro (Eds.), *Examining Developments and Applications of Wearable Devices in Modern Society* (pp. 107–133). Hershey, PA: IGI Global. doi:10.4018/978-1-5225-3290-3.ch005

Khazanchi, P., & Khazanchi, R. (2019). Hands-On Activities to Keep Students With Disabilities Engaged in K-12 Classrooms. In S. Ikuta (Ed.), *Handmade Teaching Materials for Students With Disabilities* (pp. 185–211). Hershey, PA: IGI Global. doi:10.4018/978-1-5225-6240-5.ch008

Koreeda, K., Nemoto, F., & Yamazaki, M. (2019). Focusing on the Current State of Special Needs Education in Japan and the Utilization of Handmade Teaching Materials. In S. Ikuta (Ed.), *Handmade Teaching Materials for Students With Disabilities* (pp. 20–48). Hershey, PA: IGI Global. doi:10.4018/978-1-5225-6240-5.ch002

Mattos, É. B., Guimarães, I. M., Gonçalves da Silva, A., Barreto, C. M., & Teixeira, G. A. (2016). Smart Device Clickers: Learning Basic Sciences and Biotechnology. In J. Holland (Ed.), *Wearable Technology and Mobile Innovations for Next-Generation Education* (pp. 295–320). Hershey, PA: IGI Global. doi:10.4018/978-1-5225-0069-8.ch015

McCartney, J. L. (2018). Demystifying Deafness: Helpful Information for Classroom Teachers. In P. Epler (Ed.), *Instructional Strategies in General Education and Putting the Individuals With Disabilities Act (IDEA) Into Practice* (pp. 93–131). Hershey, PA: IGI Global. doi:10.4018/978-1-5225-3111-1.ch004

McGlynn-Stewart, M., MacKay, T., Gouweleeuw, B., Hobman, L., Maguire, N., Mogyorodi, E., & Ni, V. (2017). Toys or Tools?: Educators' Use of Tablet Applications to Empower Young Students Through Open-Ended Literacy Learning. In M. Mills & D. Wake (Eds.), *Empowering Learners With Mobile Open-Access Learning Initiatives* (pp. 74–96). Hershey, PA: IGI Global. doi:10.4018/978-1-5225-2122-8.ch006

Mehdi, M., & Alharby, A. (2016). Purpose, Scope, and Technical Considerations of Wearable Technologies. In J. Holland (Ed.), *Wearable Technology and Mobile Innovations for Next-Generation Education* (pp. 1–19). Hershey, PA: IGI Global. doi:10.4018/978-1-5225-0069-8.ch001

Mkrttchian, V. (2018). Project-Based Learning for Students With Intellectual Disabilities. In P. Epler (Ed.), *Instructional Strategies in General Education and Putting the Individuals With Disabilities Act (IDEA) Into Practice* (pp. 196–221). Hershey, PA: IGI Global. doi:10.4018/978-1-5225-3111-1.ch007

Neto, J. S., Silva, A. L., Nakano, F., Pérez-Álcazar, J. J., & Kofuji, S. T. (2018). When Wearable Computing Meets Smart Cities: Assistive Technology Empowering Persons With Disabilities. In S. Delabrida Silva, R. Rabelo Oliveira, & A. Loureiro (Eds.), *Examining Developments and Applications of Wearable Devices in Modern Society* (pp. 58–85). Hershey, PA: IGI Global. doi:10.4018/978-1-5225-3290-3.ch003

Nishimura, T., & Doi, K. (2019). Easily Readable Braille Pattern for Reading Beginners and Variable Size Braille Printing System. In S. Ikuta (Ed.), *Handmade Teaching Materials for Students With Disabilities* (pp. 338–354). Hershey, PA: IGI Global. doi:10.4018/978-1-5225-6240-5.ch015

Njeru, M. W. (2017). Mobile Open-Access Revolutionizing Learning Among University Students in Kenya: The Role of the Smartphone. In M. Mills & D. Wake (Eds.), *Empowering Learners With Mobile Open-Access Learning Initiatives* (pp. 144–165). Hershey, PA: IGI Global. doi:10.4018/978-1-5225-2122-8.ch009

Obonyo, C. N. (2019). Preparing Preservice Teachers to Use Mobile Technologies. In A. Forkosh Baruch & H. Meishar Tal (Eds.), *Mobile Technologies in Educational Organizations* (pp. 42–62). Hershey, PA: IGI Global. doi:10.4018/978-1-5225-8106-2.ch003

Okawara, H., Koyama, T., Shiraishi, T., Ishida, S., Shingu, C., & Okawara, A. (2019). Development of Teaching Materials to Support Learning of Children With Cerebral Palsy in the Japanese Curriculum: Japan School Initiatives. In S. Ikuta (Ed.), *Handmade Teaching Materials for Students With Disabilities* (pp. 160–184). Hershey, PA: IGI Global. doi:10.4018/978-1-5225-6240-5.ch007

Onodipe, G. O. (2017). Engaging and Empowering Dual Enrollment Students: A Principles of Economics Course Example. In M. Mills & D. Wake (Eds.), *Empowering Learners With Mobile Open-Access Learning Initiatives* (pp. 167–192). Hershey, PA: IGI Global. doi:10.4018/978-1-5225-2122-8.ch010

Paris, D. G., & Miller, K. R. (2016). Wearables and People with Disabilities: Socio-Cultural and Vocational Implications. In J. Holland (Ed.), *Wearable Technology and Mobile Innovations for Next-Generation Education* (pp. 167–183). Hershey, PA: IGI Global. doi:10.4018/978-1-5225-0069-8.ch009

Perez, L., Gulley, A., & Prickett, L. (2017). Improving Access to Higher Education With UDL and Switch Access Technology: A Case Study. In M. Mills & D. Wake (Eds.), *Empowering Learners With Mobile Open-Access Learning Initiatives* (pp. 13–30). Hershey, PA: IGI Global. doi:10.4018/978-1-5225-2122-8.ch002

Prescott, J., Iliff, P., Edmondson, D. J., & Cross, D. (2019). Students as Co-Creators of a Mobile App to Enhance Learning and Teaching in HE. In A. Forkosh Baruch & H. Meishar Tal (Eds.), *Mobile Technologies in Educational Organizations* (pp. 96–116). Hershey, PA: IGI Global. doi:10.4018/978-1-5225-8106-2.ch006

Ragonis, N., & Dagan, O. (2019). Enhance Active Learning in Higher Education by Using Mobile Learning. In A. Forkosh Baruch & H. Meishar Tal (Eds.), *Mobile Technologies in Educational Organizations* (pp. 15–41). Hershey, PA: IGI Global. doi:10.4018/978-1-5225-8106-2.ch002

Ribeiro, J. (2016). Wearable Technology Spending: A Strategic Approach to Decision-Making. In J. Holland (Ed.), *Wearable Technology and Mobile Innovations for Next-Generation Education* (pp. 37–57). Hershey, PA: IGI Global. doi:10.4018/978-1-5225-0069-8.ch003

Seifert, T., & Zimon, V. (2019). Using Tablet Applications as Assistive Tools in Teaching English as a Foreign Language. In A. Forkosh Baruch & H. Meishar Tal (Eds.), *Mobile Technologies in Educational Organizations* (pp. 263–282). Hershey, PA: IGI Global. doi:10.4018/978-1-5225-8106-2.ch013

Silva, A. D., Rigo, S. J., & Barbosa, J. L. (2018). Wearable Health Care Ubiquitous System for Stroke Monitoring and Alert. In S. Delabrida Silva, R. Rabelo Oliveira, & A. Loureiro (Eds.), *Examining Developments and Applications of Wearable Devices in Modern Society* (pp. 134–160). Hershey, PA: IGI Global. doi:10.4018/978-1-5225-3290-3.ch006

Silva, I., Silva, K. N., Lotthammer, K. S., Bilessimo, S., & Silva, J. B. (2019). Social Innovation in Public Schools: A Case Study on the Remote Experimentation Laboratory of the Federal University of Santa Catarina. In A. Forkosh Baruch & H. Meishar Tal (Eds.), *Mobile Technologies in Educational Organizations* (pp. 1–14). Hershey, PA: IGI Global. doi:10.4018/978-1-5225-8106-2.ch001

Smith, S. (2017). Mobile Makerspace Carts: A Practical Model to Transcend Access and Space. In M. Mills & D. Wake (Eds.), *Empowering Learners With Mobile Open-Access Learning Initiatives* (pp. 31–46). Hershey, PA: IGI Global. doi:10.4018/978-1-5225-2122-8.ch004

Tal, H. M. (2019). Strategies for Developing Mobile Location-Based Learning Activities by Teachers. In A. Forkosh Baruch & H. Meishar Tal (Eds.), *Mobile Technologies in Educational Organizations* (pp. 85–95). Hershey, PA: IGI Global. doi:10.4018/978-1-5225-8106-2.ch005

Tatematsu, E. (2019). Effects of Tangible Teaching Materials According to Evaluation of Cognitive Development. In S. Ikuta (Ed.), *Handmade Teaching Materials for Students With Disabilities* (pp. 132–159). Hershey, PA: IGI Global. doi:10.4018/978-1-5225-6240-5.ch006

Torres, M. L., & Ramos, V. J. (2018). Music Therapy: A Pedagogical Alternative for ASD and ID Students in Regular Classrooms. In P. Epler (Ed.), *Instructional Strategies in General Education and Putting the Individuals With Disabilities Act (IDEA) Into Practice* (pp. 222–244). Hershey, PA: IGI Global. doi:10.4018/978-1-5225-3111-1.ch008

Trumble, J., Farah, Y. N., & Slykhuis, D. A. (2017). Teaching Exceptional Children With Mobile Technologies in a General Education Classroom. In M. Mills & D. Wake (Eds.), *Empowering Learners With Mobile Open-Access Learning Initiatives* (pp. 263–287). Hershey, PA: IGI Global. doi:10.4018/978-1-5225-2122-8.ch014

Vasconcelos, S. V., & Balula, A. (2017). Socrative: Using Mobile Devices to Promote Language Learning. In M. Mills & D. Wake (Eds.), *Empowering Learners With Mobile Open-Access Learning Initiatives* (pp. 215–237). Hershey, PA: IGI Global. doi:10.4018/978-1-5225-2122-8.ch012

Vigilante, R. J. Jr, & Hoile, M. B. (2018). Assistive Technology for the General Education Classroom. In P. Epler (Ed.), *Instructional Strategies in General Education and Putting the Individuals With Disabilities Act (IDEA) Into Practice* (pp. 132–166). Hershey, PA: IGI Global. doi:10.4018/978-1-5225-3111-1.ch005

Related Readings

Vuković, M., Car, Ž., Pavlisa, J. I., & Mandić, L. (2018). Smartwatch as an Assistive Technology: Tracking System for Detecting Irregular User Movement. _International Journal of E-Health and Medical Communications_, _9_(1), 23–34. doi:10.4018/IJEHMC.2018010102

Watanabe, D. (2016). The ScavengAR Hunt: An Augmented Reality Teacher Training Case Study Using Mobile Devices. In J. Holland (Ed.), _Wearable Technology and Mobile Innovations for Next-Generation Education_ (pp. 224–246). Hershey, PA: IGI Global. doi:10.4018/978-1-5225-0069-8.ch012

Woolman, T. A. (2016). Trends in Wearable Technologies for Earth Science. In J. Holland (Ed.), _Wearable Technology and Mobile Innovations for Next-Generation Education_ (pp. 248–268). Hershey, PA: IGI Global. doi:10.4018/978-1-5225-0069-8.ch013

Xiu, Y., Fulgencio, J. L., Asino, T. I., & Baker, A. D. (2017). Mobile Apps in Open Educational Resources. In M. Mills & D. Wake (Eds.), _Empowering Learners With Mobile Open-Access Learning Initiatives_ (pp. 120–143). Hershey, PA: IGI Global. doi:10.4018/978-1-5225-2122-8.ch008

Yang, Z., & Ganz, A. (2017). Egocentric Landmark-Based Indoor Guidance System for the Visually Impaired. _International Journal of E-Health and Medical Communications_, _8_(3), 55–69. doi:10.4018/IJEHMC.2017070104

Zilka, G. C. (2019). The Use of Mobile Technologies by Immigrant Adolescents in Coping With the New Language and With Their Formal Studies. In A. Forkosh Baruch & H. Meishar Tal (Eds.), _Mobile Technologies in Educational Organizations_ (pp. 192–209). Hershey, PA: IGI Global. doi:10.4018/978-1-5225-8106-2.ch010

About the Contributors

Teresita de Jesús Álvarez Robles is a prominent last year student of Inter-institutional Ph.D. in Computer Science held by the Universidad Veracruzana in Mexico. Her main research topic focuses on User-eXperience, Usability, HCI, Interactive Mobile Systems for blind users, in both Software Engineering and Augmented Reality (AR). She has extended her research across Mexican territory; enriching it with congress presentations and books chapters in Brazil, Chile, Costa Rica and Spain.

Francisco Álvarez Rodríguez is a Professor of Software Engineering. He holds a BA. in Informatics (1994) and an MA. (1997) from the Autonomous University of Aguascalientes and an EdD degree from the Education Institute of Tamaulipas, México and he is Ph.D. from the National Autonomous University of Mexico. He has published research papers in several international conferences in the topics of software engineering and e-learning process. His research interests are software engineering lifecycles for small and medium-sized enterprises and software engineering process for e-learning. He is currently president of the National Council for Accreditation of programs and Computing, A.C. (CONAIC).

Edgard Benítez-Guerrero is a Full-Time Professor at the Faculty of Statistics and Informatics at the Universidad Veracruzana in Mexico. He holds a PhD in Computer Science from the Université Joseph Fourier (Grenoble-I) in France, a Diplôme d'Etudes Approfondies en Informatique: Systèmes et Communications from the same university, and a M. Sc. in Artificial Intelligence from the Universidad Veracruzana, Mexico. His research interests focus on Ambient Intelligence, Human-Computer Interaction, Databases and CSCW with applications to Education and Decision Making.

* * *

Ana Antunes is a Graduate in Psychology from the Faculty of Psychology and Educational Sciences of Lisbon, Master in Human Resource Development Policies and PhD in Psychology from the University Institute of Lisbon (ISCTE-IUL). Adjunct Professor at the Superior School of Social Communication - Instituto Politécnico de Lisboa. Sub-coordinator of the Master's degree in Advertising and Marketing of this School (Superior School of Social Communication). Author of several national and international publications, her current research interests include positive organizational behavior, social media engagement, and technology and user experience issues.

Juana Canul-Reich received the Ph.D. degree in computer science and engineering from the University of South Florida in 2010. She is a Fulbrighter. She is currently a Faculty Member with the Academic Division of Informatics and Systems, Universidad Juárez Autónoma de Tabasco, México, where she is a Graduate Advisor of master and Ph.D. students. Her research interests include data mining and machine learning with the focus on microarray data analysis, medical data analysis, and seismic data analysis, and performance evaluation of algorithms. Mainly interested in problems of dimensionality reduction, classification, data exploration, preprocessing, and visualization. In 2015, she received the membership of the National System of Researchers level 1 (SNI 1) in México. She is an active reviewer for the Journal of Ambient Intelligence and Smart Environments, for Sinectica -a Mexican Journal in Education, and for diverse international conferences.

Juan Pedro Cardona Salas is a full-time professor at Universidad Autónoma de Aguascalientes (UAA) in Aguascalientes, México. Has a degree in Pedagogy, His research topics are in software engineer, Learning Object Technology, cloud computing and knowledge management.

Carolina López-Suero is professor in the Department of Chemical, Industrial and Food Engineering at Universidad Iberoamericana, since 2013. From 2016 to date, she is the Chief of the Departmental Chemistry Service. She received a B.S. in Chemistry from Universidad Nacional Autónoma de México in 1999 and a Ph.D. in Chemistry from the same university in 2004. From 2010 to 2013, she was the Chief of Sustainable Development Engineering at Instituto Tecnológico y de Estudios Superiores de Monterrey, Campus Santa Fe, Mexico. In previous years, she worked in several projects with the Mexican industry. Her research interests are green chemistry, sustainability and inclusive science-education. She has published different books and papers in these fields. She is member of the Mexican Centre of Microscale and Green Chemistry. She was Mexico's academic representative in international meetings organized by the Organization for the Prohibition of Chemical Weapons in Holland and Argentina in 2014.

Martín Montes Rivera was born in Mexico City, he studied Mechatronic Engineering and Control and Automation Engineering Maestry at Universidad Politécnica de Aguascalientes, he worked in Mechatronic Engineering Departent at Universidad Politécnica de Aguascalientes from 2014 to 2015 and he has worked in the Research and Posgrades department of Universidad Politécnica de Aguascalientes from 2015 to nowadays and studies a PhD in Computer Sciences focus at Artificial Intelligence in Universidad Juárez Autónoma de Tabasco.

Jaime Muñoz-Arteaga is a full-time professor at Universidad Autónoma de Aguascalientes (UAA) in Aguascalientes, Mexico. His research topics are in the domain of human-computer interaction, e-learning and web engineering. He has published two books in Software Engineering, one book in Human-Computer Interaction and two books about Learning Object Technology.

Julio Cesar Ponce Gallegos received the B.S. degree in computer system engineering from the Universidad Autónoma de Aguascalientes(UAA) in 2003, M.S. degree in computer sciences from the UAA in 2007. and the PHD degree computer sciences from the UAA in 2010. He is currently an Professor in the Universidad Autónoma de Aguascalientes. His research interests include Evolutionary Computation, Artificial Intelligence, Educational Technology and Data Mining.

Cristina G. Reynaga-Peña is a researcher at the School of Humanities and Education at Tecnológico de Monterrey, Campus Monterrey. She obtained a PhD in Genetics from the University of California, Riverside (USA), where she studied fungal growth and morphogenesis. She has published research in the field of fungal and plant biology. She currently focuses her research on science education and teacher professional development for science teaching, with special focus on inclusion of students with visual impairment. Author of 27 papers and book chapters, 1 book and 24 patents, her production has over 1800 literature citations. She belongs to the National Research System (SNI) of CONACYT México.

Camila Silva is a Master in Audiovisual and Multimedia by Escola Superior de Comunicação Social - Instituto Politécnico de Lisboa. Her current research interest are mobile applications guidelines for the blind and digital communication.

Aurora Torres Soto graduated as a PhD in Computer Science, Systems and Information with emphasis on Artificial Intelligence at the Autonomous University of Aguascalientes, Mexico, in 2010. She completed her Master's degree in Informatics and Computational Technologies in 2001. She studied Electronic Engineering at the Technological Institute of San Luis Potosí and she received her B.A. degree in 1994. Her areas of interest are evolvable hardware, machine learning, metaheuristics and medical and social assistance intelligent systems. She is coordinator of intelligence computing engineering at the Aguascalientes Autonomous University He is a full-time professor assigned to the Computational Sciences Department. She has worked as a professor and researcher at the Autonomous University of Aguascalientes since 1998.

César Eduardo Velázquez Amador is a full-time professor at Universidad Autónoma de Aguascalientes (UAA) in Aguascalientes, México. He was graduated as a PhD. in Exact Sciences, Systems and the Information with emphasis on Software Engineering. His research topics are in the domain of Learning Technologies, E-learning, Service Theory, Software Engineering and Information Technology Adoption. He has published papers and chapters books about learning object quality assessment and the Service Theory integration in learning technologies.

Index

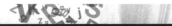
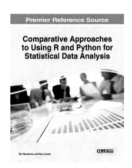
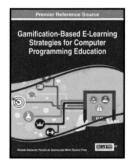
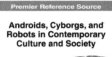
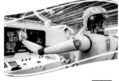
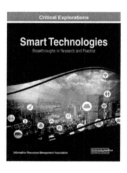
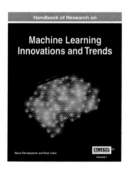
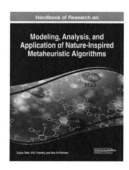
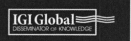

Ensure Quality Research is Introduced to the Academic Community

Become an IGI Global Reviewer for Authored Book Projects

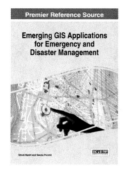

Premier Reference Source

Emerging GIS Applications for Emergency and Disaster Management

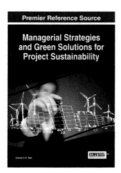

Premier Reference Source

Managerial Strategies and Green Solutions for Project Sustainability

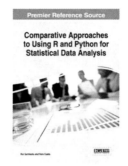

Premier Reference Source

Comparative Approaches to Using R and Python for Statistical Data Analysis

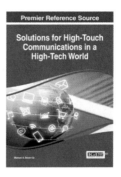

Premier Reference Source

Solutions for High-Touch Communications in a High-Tech World

The overall success of an authored book project is dependent on quality and timely reviews.

In this competitive age of scholarly publishing, constructive and timely feedback significantly expedites the turnaround time of manuscripts from submission to acceptance, allowing the publication and discovery of forward-thinking research at a much more expeditious rate. Several IGI Global authored book projects are currently seeking highly qualified experts in the field to fill vacancies on their respective editorial review boards:

Applications may be sent to:
development@igi-global.com

Applicants must have a doctorate (or an equivalent degree) as well as publishing and reviewing experience. Reviewers are asked to write reviews in a timely, collegial, and constructive manner. All reviewers will begin their role on an ad-hoc basis for a period of one year, and upon successful completion of this term can be considered for full editorial review board status, with the potential for a subsequent promotion to Associate Editor.

If you have a colleague that may be interested in this opportunity, we encourage you to share this information with them.

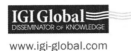

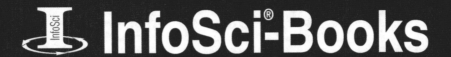
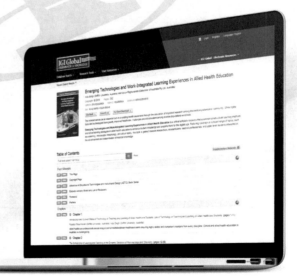

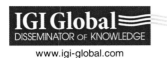 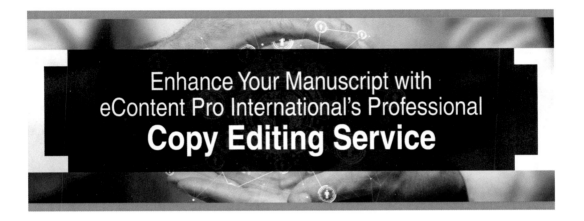

Printed in the United States
By Bookmasters